Praise for *Nursing Ethics in Everyday Practice*

"The drama of nursing lies not on the front pages of The New York Times, *but in everyday encounters with patients and families of the tiniest and sickest babies, of heartbreaking decisions bringing closure on life-extending treatment, and balancing the resources of time and staff against the realities of costs and quality. Dr. Ulrich and her colleagues bring this and more into exceptional focus for the practicing nurse."*

–Neville E. Strumpf, PhD, RN, FAAN
Professor, School of Nursing
University of Pennsylvania

*"*Nursing Ethics in Everyday Practice *provides insightful and easy-to-grasp tips to resolve ethically difficult situations at the bedside. It will be helpful for any nurse who wants to learn more about ethical issues that complicate our practice."*

–Garrett Chan, PhD, APRN, FAEN, FPCN, FAAN
Associate Adjunct Professor, Department of Physiological Nursing
University of California, San Francisco

"Connie Ulrich is a national leader on nursing ethics, and her expertise, wisdom, and empathy show on every page of Nursing Ethics in Everyday Practice. *There is no better guide to the ethical challenges of day-to-day nursing practice."*

–Arthur Caplan
Professor of Medical Ethics
Department of Medical Ethics and Health Policy
University of Pennsylvania

Nursing Ethics in Everyday Practice

Edited by Connie M. Ulrich, PhD, RN, FAAN

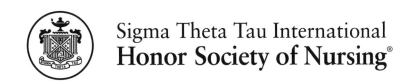

Sigma Theta Tau International
Honor Society of Nursing®

Copyright © 2012 by Sigma Theta Tau International

The Honor Society of Nursing, Sigma Theta Tau International (STTI) is a nonprofit organization whose mission is to support the learning, knowledge, and professional development of nurses committed to making a difference in health worldwide. Founded in 1922, STTI has 130,000 members in 86 countries. Members include practicing nurses, instructors, researchers, policymakers, entrepreneurs and others. STTI's 482 chapters are located at 626 institutions of higher education throughout Australia, Botswana, Brazil, Canada, Colombia, Ghana, Hong Kong, Japan, Kenya, Malawi, Mexico, the Netherlands, Pakistan, Portugal, Singapore, South Africa, South Korea, Swaziland, Sweden, Taiwan, Tanzania, United Kingdom, United States, and Wales. More information about STTI can be found online at www.nursingsociety.org.

Sigma Theta Tau International
550 West North Street
Indianapolis, IN, USA 46202

To order additional books, buy in bulk, or order for corporate use, contact Nursing Knowledge International at 888. NKI.4YOU (888.654.4968/US and Canada) or +1.317.634.8171 (outside US and Canada).

To request a review copy for course adoption, e-mail solutions@nursingknowledge.org or call 888.NKI.4YOU (888.654.4968/US and Canada) or +1.317.634.8171 (outside US and Canada).

To request author information, or for speaker or other media requests, contact Rachael McLaughlin of the Honor Society of Nursing, Sigma Theta Tau International at 888.634.7575 (US and Canada) or +1.317.634.8171 (outside US and Canada).

ISBN: 9781935476504
EPUB ISBN: 9781935476511
MOBI ISBN: 9781937554255
PDF ISBN: 9781935476528

Library of Congress Cataloging-in-Publication Data

Ulrich, Connie M., 1960-
 Nursing ethics in everyday practice : a step-by-step guide / Connie M. Ulrich.
    p. ; cm.
 Includes bibliographical references.
 ISBN 978-1-935476-50-4 (alk. paper)
 I. Sigma Theta Tau International. II. Title.
 [DNLM: 1. Ethics, Nursing. 2. Nursing Care--methods. WY 85]

 174.2'9--dc23
                    2011047112

First Printing, 2012

Publisher: Renee Wilmeth

Acquisitions Editors: Janet Boivin and Emily Hatch

Editorial Coordinator: Paula Jeffers

Cover Designer: Michael Tanamachi

Interior Design and Page Composition: Rebecca Batchelor

Principal Editor: Carla Hall

Development Editor: Amy Moshier

Copy Editor: Kevin Kent

Proofreader: Barbara Bennett

Indexer: Johnna Van Hoose Dinse

Dedication

To Keith E. Ulrich, with gratitude for his love of ethical discourse

To Dr. Karen Soeken, professor emeritus, University of Maryland, Baltimore, whose dedicated teaching and student mentorship started my path of bioethics-related inquiry

Acknowledgements

I would like to acknowledge the assistance of Carla Hall, Emily Hatch, and Janet Boivin at Sigma Theta Tau International for their discussions surrounding the need for this book, and their interest in the everyday ethical issues that bedside nurses are facing. I would also like to thank all of the chapter contributors for their expertise and willingness to share their knowledge with practicing nurses. I owe a special note of gratitude to Dr. Christine Grady for writing the foreword in this book and for her continuing guidance on ethics-related issues in nursing practice and research. I would also like to thank Dr. Sarah Kagan and the Society of Otorhinolaryngology and Head-Neck Nurses for inviting me to share some of my concerns related to ethical issues in nursing, which is why this book came about. A note of thanks to my sister, Theresa Hixson, for her encouragement, laughter, and assistance in moving this book forward. And finally, I would like to thank my many students who have openly discussed the need for ethics training and willingly shared their insights.

About the Author

Connie Ulrich is an associate professor of bioethics and nursing at the University of Pennsylvania School of Nursing with a secondary appointment in the Department of Medical Ethics and Health Policy in the School of Medicine. Ulrich received a diploma in nursing from the Williamsport Hospital School of Nursing, a bachelor's and master's degree in nursing from the Catholic University of America, and a doctoral degree from the University of Maryland, Baltimore, with a concentration in nursing ethics. Ulrich has published on bioethics topics in both nursing and medicine. She is a fellow of the American Academy of Nursing.

About the Contributing Authors

Karen Baker, MSN, CRNP

Karen Baker is a nurse practitioner at the National Institutes of Health. She participated in the development of the Pain and Palliative Care Service and continues to work there as a clinician. She is a faculty member for the Hospice and Palliative Care Fellowship program at NIH. In addition to her clinical nursing work, she frequently teaches clinical symptom management and participates as an associate investigator on clinical trials exploring palliative care issues.

Marna S. Barrett, PhD

Marna S. Barrett joined the faculty of the University of Pennsylvania School of Medicine, Department of Psychiatry, in 2001. A 1993 graduate of the University of Memphis, Barrett is a licensed clinical psychologist, a certified genetic counselor, and a diplomat of the American Board of Medical Genetics. She is a member of the advisory board of The Scattergood Program for the Applied Ethics of Behavioral Healthcare. Barrett's research focuses on psychotherapy, attrition, and mood disorders. She has authored or co-authored more than 25 publications, has presented her research nationally and internationally, and regularly provides workshops on ethics and ethical decision-making in mental health. She is a clinical associate professor of psychology and director of research studies in the Mood and Anxiety Disorders Treatment and Research Center in the Department of Psychiatry at the University of Pennsylvania and teaches the Department of Psychiatry's ethics curriculum for the residency program. She maintains a clinical practice focused on the treatment of depression and bipolar disorder.

Kathleen Calzone, PhD, RN, APNG, FAAN

Kathleen Calzone is a senior nurse specialist for research in the Genetics branch of the Center for Cancer Research at the National Cancer Institute, National Institutes of Health. Calzone is credentialed in genetics by the Genetic Nursing Credentialing Commission and is a past president of the International Society of Nurses in Genetics. She co-edited the book *Genetics and Genomics in Oncology Nursing Practice*. She has published extensively and presented her work both nationally and internationally.

Margaret Cotroneo, PhD, PMHCNS-BC

Margaret Cotroneo is associate professor emerita of psychiatric mental health nursing at the University of Pennsylvania School of Nursing. Her work has centered on teaching and studying the interface of families, systems, and health, with a focus on relational dynamics, for more than 40 years. Formerly, she directed the School of Nursing's psychiatric-mental health program. She also served as faculty director of the School of Nursing's nurse-managed community health center, unique for its pioneering integration of primary care and behavioral health in the nursing center model. A practicing family therapist, she held a secondary appointment with the University of Pennsylvania School of Medicine's Department of Psychiatry and later co-directed the University of Pennsylvania's cross-disciplinary Master of Science in Public Health program. She has taught and published internationally and was awarded a Fulbright professorship to Germany.

Elizabeth Gingell Epstein, PhD, RN

Elizabeth Gingell Epstein is an assistant professor of nursing at the University of Virginia School of Nursing and a faculty affiliate in the Center for Biomedical Ethics and Humanities at the University of Virginia. She is a member of the Ethics Consult Service and the Ethics Committee, and she coordinates the Moral Distress Consult Service for the University of Virginia Health System. Epstein's research focuses on ethical issues that arise in neonatal and pediatric intensive care.

Michele Mathes, JD

Michele Mathes is director of education at the Center for Advocacy for the Rights and Interests of the Elderly (CARIE). She serves as adjunct faculty at Drexel University College of Medicine, St. Joseph's University Institute of Catholic Bioethics, and is a member of the advisory board of the College of Health Sciences of Salus University. She has co-authored a number of articles, including "Competence with Compassion: Ethical Decision-Making in Long Term Care," "Commitment, Relationship, Voice: Cornerstones for an Ethics of Long-Term Care," and "Compliance with Advance Directives: Wrongful Living and Tort Law Incentives."

Kim Moony-Doyle, MSN, RN

Kim Mooney-Doyle, CPNP, CPON, is a doctoral candidate at the University of Pennsylvania School of Nursing. She has received federal funding to study parenting in the context of pediatric palliative care. While the majority of her career has included clinical practice, education, and research in pediatric oncology, she has worked both nationally and internationally in public health and community health.

Freida Hopkins Outlaw, PhD, RN, FAAN

Freida Hopkins Outlaw is a graduate of Berea College and Boston College. She is developing an adolescent health and wellness center for Meharry Medical College. Formerly, she was assistant commissioner, Division of Special Populations and Minority Services, and chief nurse for five regional mental health institutes with the Tennessee Department of Mental Health and Developmental Disabilities. While in this position, she was awarded more than $32 million in federally competitive grants. Outlaw has published more than 20 manuscripts and book chapters and has presented on various aspects of health and mental health, with a focus on children, youth, and their families.

June Roman, MSN, RN, PMHCNS-BC

June Roman is associate course director for the undergraduate nursing program at the University of Pennsylvania School of Nursing and site coordinator for the graduate nurse practitioner clinical practicum. She has taught in the undergraduate and graduate programs since 2008. She has worked as a clinician in psychiatric nursing for more than 42 years, including inpatient settings, home care, consultation, and private counseling. She has presented and published in research related to HIV and the serious mentally ill.

Fiona Timmins, PhD, MSc, BNS RNT, FFNRCSI, BSc Health & Soc (Open)

Fiona Timmons is senior lecturer and associate professor for the School of Nursing and Midwifery, Trinity College Dublin. She has authored more than 65 publications in peer-reviewed journals and has authored or co-authored six nursing textbooks. She is a reviewer for several peer-reviewed journals and serves on a number of editorial boards. Her research interests include professional nursing issues, nurse education, spirituality, and reflection.

Gwenyth R. Wallen, PhD, RN

Gwenyth R. Wallen is chief of nursing research and translational science at the National Institutes of Health, Clinical Center. Her clinical research focuses on pain and symptom measurement in the context of chronic disease management and at the end of life. She has served as a scientific member of the institutional review board for the Eunice Kennedy Shriver National Institute of Child Health and Human Development since 2001.

Mary K. Walton, MSN, MBE, RN

Mary K. Walton is a nurse ethicist, the director of patient/family centered care at the Hospital of the University of Pennsylvania, and an associate fellow of the University of Pennsylvania Center for Bioethics. She has practiced in academic health care settings for more than 35 years and has a progressive history of leadership. Past roles of clinical nurse specialist and nurse manager included responsibility for clinical ethics committees, ethics consultation services, cultural competency training, and evidence-based practice standards. She is responsible for organizational initiatives focused on clinical ethics and improving the patient and family experience of care. She has published in the areas of collaboration, advocacy, healthy work environment, nursing history, and patient-centered care.

Lucia D. Wocial, PhD, RN

Lucia D. Wocial is nurse ethicist and program leader in the Fairbanks Program in Nursing Ethics at Indiana University Health and adjunct assistant professor at the Indiana University School of Nursing, Department of Family Health. She practiced neonatal intensive care nursing for more than 25 years, including 10 years as a certified neonatal clinical nurse specialist. She has extensive experience consulting on clinical ethics and has published several articles in peer-reviewed journals. She has spoken at local, regional, national, and international conferences on topics related to neonatal nursing and ethics. Her area of research is moral distress of professional caregivers.

Mindy Zeitzer, PhD, MBE, RN

Mindy Zeitzer received her PhD in nursing and ethics in 2009 and her master's in bioethics in 2008, both degrees from the University of Pennsylvania. She received her Master of Science in Nursing as an acute care nurse practitioner in 2004. Her clinical background is in intensive care, where she worked with cardiothoracic and trauma/surgical patients. Her research focuses on ethical issues encountered by nurses in acute care and emergency settings. She maintains an adjunct professorship position at Thomas Jefferson University.

Table of Contents

Foreword

Nurses everywhere encounter ethical issues in their practice. Nurses make everyday decisions about the form and content of communication with patients and families—how to balance compassion and direction; make recommendations and promote autonomous treatment authorization; allocate their time, energy, and available resources; soothe pain and suffering; and optimize their patients' well-being and protect their rights. Evolving changes in our health care system, changes in the demographics of ill and hospitalized patients, emerging technologies, cost constraints, and an aging provider workforce continue to present novel and complex ethical challenges for nurses. Unfortunately, nurses have often felt uncomfortable or unprepared to address the ethical challenges they face in their practice. When nurses are given adequate tools, education, and support to recognize the ubiquitous everyday ethical challenges and to confidently seek strategies and solutions to address them—often in collaboration with their professional colleagues—their voices resonate with commitment, courage, and resourcefulness. All of us are the beneficiaries.

Connie Ulrich notes in this volume that nurses' voices are among the strongest assets in our current health care system. Dr. Ulrich herself continues to be an influential and unwavering voice for the ethical practice of nursing. In her invaluable work, she studies and advocates for ethics education for nurses, ethics resources and environments that support ethical nursing practice, and strategies for empowering nurses to provide the highest quality ethical care to their patients. She has documented that the stress nurses often feel when they lack the confidence or ability to address ethical tensions in their work can lead to moral distress and to dissatisfaction with their jobs and the profession.

This book adds to Dr. Ulrich's growing collection of contributions promoting the ethical practice of nursing by providing information and guidance about everyday ethics for nurses practicing on the front lines. In this volume, she has gathered the sage voices of leaders in nursing ethics in a collection that addresses a wide range of issues. Using complex but sometimes familiar case examples, the contributors guide readers to recognize ethical issues in nursing care, and to systematically use ethical principles, codes and standards, precedent, and careful thought to identify promising courses of action and responses to complex situations. The book provides readers with models of ethical decision making and overarching guidance regarding communication and moral courage. Dr. Ulrich and her contributors draw particular attention to ethical challenges in various sub-specialties, including acute care, long-term care, palliative care, neonatal care, pediatric care, and psychiatric care. Ethical considerations in clinical research and in genetics provide additional breadth to the book's coverage. The result is a welcome and useful guide for nurses as they develop their professional moral compass, exercise their moral agency, effectively utilize ethics resources, and confidently navigate the sometimes thorny terrain of ethical nursing practice in the interests of the patients and communities they serve.

Thanks to the work of Connie Ulrich and her colleagues, ethically informed practice can be a signature strength demonstrated through the voices and actions of practicing nurses.

–Christine Grady, PhD, RN
Chair, Department of Bioethics
National Institutes of Health Clinical Center

Introduction

"You gain strength, courage, and confidence by every experience in which you really stop to look fear in the face. You are able to say to yourself, 'I have lived through this horror. I can take the next thing that comes along.' You must do the thing you think you cannot do."

–Eleanor Roosevelt

As nurses, we face tremendous challenges and often see and do things that are extraordinary. How many of us have done things that we thought we just could not do—or do again—in health care? We could not take care of another young victim with gunshot wounds; we could not see another child abused, injured, or hurt in some way; we could not see another homeless victim with health care needs so massive that we were providing only a band-aid approach; we could not see another newly diagnosed child with bone cancer with an uncertain future—one most likely filled with physical and emotional disfigurement. Bedside nursing is one of the most challenging careers within the health care sector, yet it is also one of the most rewarding. To say it simply, it is not an easy job.

"Staff nurses," as they are commonly called, represent more than two-thirds of the United States nursing population and are employed mostly within hospitals or other health care facilities such as nursing homes (U.S. Department of Health and Human Services, Health Resources and Services Administration, 2010). Within hospital walls, however, is a host of complex human illnesses where ethical conflicts can easily occur because of power imbalances. These ethical conflicts include provider, patient, and family disputes; patient-related suffering; care path decisions; and endless opportunities for miscommunication about care delivery.

Ethical questions often arise in nursing practice because of professional obligations to "do good." Nurses want to act in the best interests of their patients, but they are sometimes challenged by competing demands, including the complexity and immediate needs of other patients as well as resource constraints. In addition, it is not always clear how to "do good" in certain situations, especially because illness is often intertwined with suffering. Broader social issues of poverty, joblessness, and other distressing economic markers challenge the health care system. According to the U.S. Census Bureau (2011), one of six Americans lives in poverty, and nearly 50 million are uninsured. This has profound consequences for the health care system and for those who are direct patient caregivers.

"While our professional codes of conduct offer guidelines for ethical practice, providing care is murkier in the real-life dramas of everyday situations" (Ulrich & Grady, 2009, p. 6).

The purpose of this book is to present some of these "murkier" ethical challenges nurses encounter in various clinical situations and assist them in finding reasonable solutions. This book is an introductory text for nurses looking for strategies and tools to better communicate with patients, families, and health care teams concerning ethical issues in practice and to lead interdisciplinary discussions for resolving bedside controversies.

Nurses face ethical issues every day. Consider, for example, caring for an emergency room patient who requires massive amounts of blood products and medications, but whose outcome seems grim. The nurse might question the appropriateness of such aggressive care and wonder if an advance directive outlines the patient's wishes for life-sustaining treatment. Which member of the health care team decides what constitutes "enough care" in this particular case? And, importantly, is this a fair and judicious use of finite resources? Think about another situation where a nurse is caring for a critically ill child diagnosed with terminal cancer whose parents refuse to give up hope, asking the physicians and nurses to "do everything" they can to help the child survive. What do bedside nurses say if patients ask for advice about participation in a research protocol?

This book sheds light on these difficult ethical questions. Case studies help orient the reader by exploring scenarios, possible actions, and potential outcomes. The first part of the book covers general and overarching aspects of ethics in nursing, starting with current and future challenges in Chapter 1. Chapter 2 moves into ethical decision-making models; Chapter 3 covers moral courage or having a "voice"; Chapter 4 is about communications in ethical situations; Chapter 5 addresses ethics consultation; Chapter 6 moves into the ethics of genetics; and Chapter 7 closes Part I with research and its ethical considerations for nurses. Part II includes Chapter 8 on critical care, Chapter 9 on long-term care, Chapter 10 on palliative care, Chapter 11 on neonatal care, Chapter 12 on pediatric care, and Chapter 13 on psychiatric care.

As nurses, our responsibilities as moral agents require us to question the benefits and burdens of aggressive care, technological advancement, and determination of quality of life. In fact, Kuhse (1997) argues that nurses fail both themselves and their patients if they continually allow role misperceptions—"physicians make decisions and nurses carry them out"—to influence nursing's agenda for the public good or to dominate public discourse. Nursing's voice remains one of its strongest assets within the health care system. We have an opportunity to use our voice for the beneficent care of patients and to intervene responsively by asking thoughtful and substantive ethical questions about their care. I hope that this book will help bedside nurses find their voices and use them confidently when addressing ethical issues in their daily practice.

–Connie Ulrich

References

Kuhse, H. (1997). *Caring: Nurses, women and ethics.* Maldon, MA: Blackwell.

Ulrich, C.M., & Grady, C. (2009). Doing "good" with limited resources: Is it good enough in the provision of quality clinical care? *Clinical Scholars Review, 2*(1), 5-7.

U.S. Census Bureau. (2011, September 13). *Income, poverty and health insurance coverage in the United States: 2010.* Retrieved from http://www.census.gov/newsroom/releases/archives/income_wealth/cb11-157.html

U.S. Department of Health and Human Services, Health Resources and Services Administration. (2010). *The registered nurse population: Initial findings from the 2008 National Sample Survey of Registered Nurses.* Washington, DC: Author.

GENERAL CONSIDERATIONS OF ETHICS IN NURSING

I

WHAT DOES THE FUTURE HOLD FOR NURSING CARE?

–Connie M. Ulrich, PhD, RN, FAAN
*Associate Professor of Bioethics and Nursing,
University of Pennsylvania School of Nursing
Secondary Appointment, Department of
Medical Ethics and Health Policy
Senior Fellow, Leonard Davis Institute for Health Economics,
NewCourtland Center for Transitions and Health*

–Kim Mooney-Doyle, MSN, RN
Doctoral candidate, University of Pennsylvania School of Nursing

Think About It!

- By 2030, those 65 and older will represent nearly 20% of the total U.S. population, requiring new models of health care delivery and a skilled workforce to meet these demands.

- Providing ethical care at the end of life will require shared decision-making between the patient and the provider and an honest dialogue about the benefits and burdens of treatment. Nurses must be part of these discussions.

- The electronic health record (EHR), as one indicator of health care reform, is a means to deliver safe, efficient, and quality patient care but it is not without ethical concerns, such as privacy, confidentiality, and ownership of data.

The current cost of health care in our society is unsustainable and creates multiple ethical issues in the financing and delivery of health care. These issues impact every practicing nurse and will continue to do so in the future. As the most populous and trusted health care professionals in the United States, nurses have tremendous potential to effect positive health change for all Americans (Jones, 2010). With such great potential, however, comes an important responsibility—to understand the significance of nursing care, how culture intersects with the care we deliver, and the potential ethical issues that might arise in health care delivery.

What will the future hold for nurses as they provide care within a constrained economic environment? As life expectations increase, individuals live longer with chronic illnesses or with the sequelae of cured life-limiting illnesses, and as state-of-the-art technology continues to develop, profound ethical questions about caring for aging and chronically ill populations will abound. Issues such as delivering high-quality care in a cost-effective manner; distributing finite resources; and discussing issues of patient and family-related suffering, burden, and quality of life will be at the forefront of nursing practice.

In this chapter, we explore three demographic and societal challenges that will not only impact how we deliver care in the future, but also have profound ethical implications for nurses: aging, end-of-life care, and technology.

Aging in an Ethnically Diverse Society

Today, we live in a society that is rapidly aging and ethnically diverse. The U.S. population is living longer and healthier in this generation than in any previous generation (Centers for Disease Control [CDC], 2007; Federal Interagency Forum on Age-Related Statistics, 2010). As people get older, the potential for physical or mental weaknesses and frailty increases. Use of health care resources also increases as more people live with chronic illnesses and seek treatment for life-threatening illnesses, or experience social, behavioral, emotional, and psychological challenges because of isolation, dementia, depression, and loss of loved ones and friends (Federal Interagency Forum on Age-Related Statistics, 2010).

The Administration on Aging estimates that one in eight Americans is 65 years or older, and by 2030 this age group will represent nearly 20% of the total U.S. population (Administration on Aging [AoA], 2011). The number of minority older individuals—the fastest growing segment of the U.S. population—is projected to be 20 million by that time (Kleyman, 2009; Thai, 2010). Ivashkov and Van Norman (2009) project that by 2050, approximately eight million people will be over 85 years old.

Most concerning is that older individuals account for more than one of three (36%) U.S. hospital admissions and almost 50% of all U.S. hospital expenditures (Landefeld, 2003). Many older adults are admitted to hospitals or other health care facilities with acute illnesses compounded by other chronic diseases that add to the complexity and cost of care. These chronic conditions can include hypertension, diabetes, memory impairment, dementia, and limitations in activities of daily living. In addition, recent research has found that hospitalized Medicare patients were more likely to suffer from medical mistakes leading to serious complications and, in some cases, even death (Associated Press, 2010).

So what does all of this mean for today's practicing nurses? Certainly the public is very trusting of the nursing profession, as it continually ranks nursing first in honesty and ethical standards of conduct (Jones, 2010). As can be seen in the case study below, working with older patients can give rise to several ethical concerns associated with their care.

Case Study 1.1

Marian is a 65-year-old female diagnosed with ocular melanoma with metastasis to the liver. She has endured multiple rounds of chemotherapy, but her disease is now resistant to all treatments and her organ systems are beginning to fail. Marian is transferred to the intensive care unit (ICU), where she is placed on dialysis and ventilator support. The attending physician expresses concerns to the family about prolonging ineffective treatments. The daughter insists that all aggressive treatments continue and refuses to give up on her mother. Marian's husband is distraught and unable to discuss Marian's care; he allows the daughter to speak on his behalf. No advance directive is available to know what Marian's wishes would have been prior to her hospital admission. The daughter asks the nurse what she should do about her mother's care.

This scenario is all too common in intensive care settings. Many ethical concerns can arise: How does the nurse determine the risk-benefit of treatment for Marian? Who should make decisions on behalf of Marian? What does it mean to be a "proxy decision-maker"? Should the daughter's wishes be respected? Who determines Marian's quality of life? Must physicians and nurses continue aggressive measures when they believe they are more harmful than beneficial?

Where does the nurse begin when she or he is faced with these daunting ethical questions? The nurse might not be sure what the best interest of the patient is, yet must continue to provide care for a patient and family who are in distress.

Health Care Workforce Issues Related to Aging

The dramatic shifts in numbers expected with the growth of the aging population will influence both the actual members of the health care workforce and the care they provide to older individuals. The health care workforce itself will age. This is evident in the aging of the nursing profession, in both nurses who provide clinical care and management and the nursing faculty who teach new generations of nurses, advanced practice nurses, and nurse researchers or scientists.

Currently, the average age for a nurse in the United States is 48 years (AACN, 2011). The aging of this particular population toward retirement age has major implications, as it will affect the number of experienced nurses available to provide care and those who serve in advanced practice roles (e.g., advanced practice nurses, nurse managers, nursing educators, faculty, and research scientists; Gabrielle, Jackson, & Mannix, 2008). In fact, it is estimated that more than 250,000 nurses will be needed by 2025 (AACN, 2011). The loss of nurses in these positions will play an important part of any future nursing shortages. For example, a shortage of nursing faculty limits the number of students who can be admitted to a school, which limits the number of nursing graduates to provide nursing care (AACN, 2011). This reduced number of nurses ultimately affects the quality and safety of nursing care provided and reduces nurses' abilities to assist individuals in reaching their goals in managing health and illness.

Potential Issues Affecting the Informed Consent Process

- Severity and type of the patient's illness or disease
- Acute or chronic illness
- Cognitive deficits (e.g., patients with developmental disabilities, temporary memory loss due to an acute event, and types of mental illnesses, such as schizophrenia)
- Symptom distress (e.g., pain, shortness of breath, nausea, fatigue)
- Educational level
- Pressures from family, friends, or others
- Age of the patient
- Medications (e.g., sedatives)
- Alterations in metabolic processes, such as hypoxemia and hypoglycemia
- Hospital environment (e.g., sleep disruption in the ICU)

Adapted from: Jairath, N., Ulrich, C. M., & Ley, C. (2005). Ethical considerations in the recruitment of research subjects from hospitalized, cardiovascular patient populations. Journal of Cardiovascular Nursing. 20(1), 56-61.

As patient care is sandwiched between an increasingly aging population and a shortage in nursing workforces, one potential risk is the lack of time to adequately communicate with aging individuals about important health care concerns. Discussing the goals and ramifications of the care they seek and obtaining fully informed consent for their participation in research or health care interventions could be a significant challenge (Ivashkov & Van Norman, 2009).

The aging population is especially vulnerable during the informed consent process because many individuals might suffer from disorders that affect their cognition (e.g., Alzheimer's disease) or their ability to communicate (e.g., hearing loss; Jairath, Ulrich, & Ley, 2005). In addition, they might be influenced by stifling social factors, such as financial limitations, family pressures, and physical dependency. How do these concerns influence the manner in which informed consent and true participation in care are sought from older individuals? Examining these questions through the four major bioethical principles (i.e., beneficence, nonmaleficence, respect for autonomy, and justice) might provide more insight into this issue. Table 1.1 illustrates how these bioethical principles can be applied to the goals of caring for an aging population.

Table 1.1   Application of Bioethical Principles to Goals of Care for an Aging Population

Ethical Principles	Goals of Care
1. Beneficence 2. Nonmaleficence	*Beneficence* • Promote the greatest good by maximizing the benefits, consistent with older individuals' stated goals and health care needs. • Clear communication patterns. • Share and elicit information in a way that is acceptable to the patient. • Allow enough time for questions and reflection on care goals. • Address health-related needs of the patient within the patient's particular culture. *Nonmaleficence* • Minimize patient burden and avoid harm. • Avoid discriminatory aging perspectives toward older patients.

Ethical Principles	Goals of Care
3. Respect for Autonomy	• Each individual is considered competent to make his or her own medical decisions unless evidence to the contrary exists.
	• Informed consent to treatment or research respects the right of patients to make decisions on their behalf. Informed consent includes the essential elements of voluntariness, disclosure of information, and competence to make decisions.
	• Research suggests that older individuals who are hospitalized want detailed information about their condition so that they can make informed health care decisions (Ivashkov & Van Norman, 2009).
4. Justice	• Health care should be provided free of bias or prejudice toward older patients.
	• Older individuals should not be automatically assumed to have worsening cognitive function just by virtue of age, but rather be assessed individually in a manner that is consistent with their abilities (Ivashkov & Van Norman, 2009).
	• Older patients should be encouraged to participate in health care decisions that best elicit their health care preferences and allow their fullest participation in the process.
	• Intensive and aggressive therapies should not be automatically withheld from older individuals based simply upon age. Rather, the intervention should be considered in light of the potential benefits and burdens it accords the person.

Technology

In this section, we explore the ethical implications of technology from two different perspectives. First, we look at the intersection of technology and advanced illness. Then we discuss the role of electronic health records (EHRs) in patient care.

Technology and Advanced Illness Care Issues

Every day nurses rely on various types of equipment and other health-related accessories to care for their patients. Indeed, advances in technology have influenced almost every aspect of modern care delivery, from vaccinations to electronic charting.

In many ways, technology is hard to separate from the delivery of health care. On any given unit, high-tech machines and monitoring systems support patients during both acute and critically ill episodes of their life. Patients are often dependent on technology to monitor their physiological status, including assisting with labored or difficult breathing, improving cardiovascular performance, or preserving kidney function. Though technology has improved the quality of life for many people, it can also be burdensome, and its use at a patient's end of life is particularly distressing for many nurses.

Unfortunately, end-of-life concerns are not likely to fade in significance. In 2009, Medicare paid more than $50 billion for expenses associated with hospital care during the last 2 months of patients' lives, and there is no clarity on whether or not this costly outlay improved the patients' quality of life (CBS News, 2010). Ethics often becomes intertwined in end-of-life issues as clinicians, patients and their families, and other involved individuals seek a common framework and language from which to assess the clinical challenges stemming from the use of technology near or at the end of life (Ferrell, 2006).

This topic is of substantial importance to nursing for a multitude of reasons. First, nurses are frequently the health care representatives closest to patients and families during technologically intensive care and intensive palliative care, in addition to being the providers and evaluators of such care. Providing this emotionally laden care can potentially lead to feelings of moral distress, burn-out, powerlessness, and anxiety. Organizations that support shared decision-making among members of the interdisciplinary health care team and that respect the voice of patients and families are crucial in preventing these consequences (Catlin et al., 2008; Gavrin, 2007; Rushton, 2006).

Such experiences and sentiments of distress are not uncommon. In fact, a study by Solomon et al. (2005) found that among nurses and physicians caring for neonates, children, and adolescents, 80% endorsed the statement "We save children who should not be saved;" 45% endorsed the statement "I have acted against my conscience;" and 50% reported "The treatments I give are overly burdensome." Similar experiences are found in the adult literature (Brazil, Kassalainen, Ploeg, & Marshall, 2010; Ferrell, 2006; Piers et al., 2011).

These findings demonstrate that many health care professionals are influenced by caring for children in technologically intensive environments in the face of ethical dilemmas and questions about the appropriateness of this kind of care. Secondly, clinicians do not suffer alone. Families are deeply affected by the eventual death of their loved one, by the symptoms and suffering experienced by their loved one near the end, and by their own communication with the team caring for their loved one (Hinds et al., 2001; Wolfe et al., 2000). In fact, their decisions surrounding end-of-life care are often influenced by their relationship with the ill family member and the clinicians caring for the patient (Hinds et al., 2001).

In addition, the death of an ill adult or child leaves family members and caregivers forever changed. For example, parents of children who died of cancer report increased levels of anxiety and depression up to 9 years after the child died (Kriecbergs, Valdimarsdottir, Onelov, Henter, & Steineck, 2004). Taken together, these research findings demonstrate that end-of-life issues are pertinent to nursing care not only at the point in which it is rendered, but also as families and clinicians survive the death of cherished patients, both in the short and long terms. These findings point to the reason nurses should be at the forefront in discussions, research, and education in palliative and end-of-life care.

Nurses can initiate discussions with other members of the team, as well as families or caregivers, about the goals of care for their patients. Because nurses might come to know patients and their family or caregivers personally throughout a course of treatment, they can offer a unique perspective on how certain interventions will look, feel, and be lived in a particular context. For example, nurses can assess if a particular intervention (e.g., oxygen) is as burdensome as the environment in which it is rendered (e.g., a hospital ward or ICU; Gillick, 2009). In addition to the intervention itself, such a perspective of considering the environment contributes greatly to dialogue that helps to shape decisions and enact a patient's and family's wishes. In addition, this perspective adds to organizational and policy considerations of which technologies are available for relieving symptoms and in which environments they might be utilized (e.g., home, school). Finally, nurses can maintain ongoing conversations with families and patients about goals of care and refinements to documents, such as advance directives. Such interventions maintain the dynamic nature, as originally intended, of these kinds of documents.

Questions nurses might ask of the health care team include the following:

- Do we know what the patient and family would want in this situation?

- Has anyone discussed end-of-life issues with the patient and family?

- Is there an advance directive that indicates what the patient would want?

- Is there an available ethics committee that can help the team decipher what is in the best interest of the patient and family?

- What are the potential benefits and burdens of a given intervention in the context of a particular individual's family, geography, culture, and overall situation?

- Is technology adding burden to the patient's condition, and what is the likelihood of improvement with the intervention?

Examples of questions nurses might ask the patient (if the patient is cognitively capable) and family or caregivers include the following:

- Is there anything you would like to discuss about your illness?

- Are you familiar with an advance directive?

- Are you familiar with palliative care and hospice?

- Is there someone who could speak on your behalf if for some reason you are not able to do so?

- If your illness progresses, what would you want done in terms of your treatment (i.e., aggressive therapy, CPR, ventilator support)?

Electronic Health Records

The electronic health record (EHR) has been a topic of considerable discussion, both in clinical and political settings, and will be an important aspect of nursing care in the future. With the passage of the American Recovery and Reinvestment Act (ARRA) and the Health Information Technology for Economic and Clinical Health Act (HITECH), the electronic health record has become mandated in federal legislation (Blumenthal & Tavenner, 2010). The ARRA demonstrated unprecedented governmental support for the EHR and led to the formation of two advisory committees that would use the input of government, clinical, public, and private stakeholders and consumers to guide the process. A substantial portion of the ARRA and all of HITECH legislation aim to facilitate adoption and meaningful use of the EHR into clinical care. HITECH ties payment through Medicare and Medicaid to achievement of health care outcomes. Specifically, HITECH will make available nearly $44,000 (via Medicare) and $63,000 (via Medicaid) per clinician to institute electronic charting (Blumenthal & Tavenner, 2010).

According to the Centers for Medicare & Medicaid Services (CMS), the EHR is "an electronic version of a patient's medical history, that is maintained by the provider over time, and may include all of the key administrative clinical data relevant to that person's care under a particular provider, including demographics, progress notes, problems, medications, vital signs, past medical history, immunizations, laboratory data, and radiology reports" (2011, para. 1). Nursing care of patients across the lifespan and across locations of care will be influenced by the introduction and implementation of EHRs. For example, the EHR offers clinicians instant access to patient information and has the potential to organize and focus nursing workflow. In addition, the EHR can offer other forms of support to nurses through decision-support aids, statistical tracking and reporting for research, and reminders for patient education and anticipatory guidance.

> *The EHR is not simply a digitized paper record. Rather, it is a compendium of clinical data in one compact form that can easily be stored and transmitted between clinicians and institutions. In addition, the EHR facilitates data management and storage of system-level data for further analysis. The EHR can include many aspects of patient care including vital signs, demographic factors such as age and gender, medical history, medications, immunizations, and other related reports. (Sade, 2010, p. 40)*

Some ethical questions associated with EHRs include the following:

- Who is ultimately responsible for reviewing and acting upon new findings or results in the record?

- How does one address issues of portability, ownership, opt-out ability, adolescent control of data, parental rights to the records of their children, and management of large data sets via a multidisciplinary panel? This panel will oversee validation and analysis of the data and provision of reliable linkage of the right patient to the right EHR (considering this is erroneously done in 5–10% of cases).

- What measures are in place for clinicians to publically report potential safety issues in the design of EHR programs? Such ability is currently hampered by a clause in many such contracts to "hold harmless" the program creators (Sittig and Singh, 2011).

- Who pays for the EHR and implements it versus who benefits from it?

  - Currently, clinicians pay in terms of implementation with decreased productivity (almost at a 10% reduction). Pediatric clinicians, in particular, must also consider the costs of "safe, secure, and verifiable access to data for more than ten years" (Sittig & Singh, 2011), because the care they provide spans long periods of time (possibly more than 18 years in children). In addition, such clinicians must also consider what will be done with their patient files at clinician retirement and who will pay for the maintenance of such storage (Sittig & Singh, 2011).

- Perhaps the most significant ethical challenges for the EHR are those related to privacy and security of sensitive health information. Specifically, the Department of Health and Human Services (DHHS) is working to address such concerns on the grand scale (Blumenthal & Tavennar, 2010).

  - Legislation through the Health Insurance Portability and Accountability Act (HIPAA), ARRA, and HITECH allows for patient access to the electronic record to have an audit trail of all disclosures of information and mandates that individuals be notified for any unauthorized use. Also required through this legislation is encryption of all health information and the prohibition of sales of the data or its unauthorized use, with penalties for any infractions. Such protections are also afforded to individually maintained EHRs, such as those through Google Health or MS HealthVault.

- The potential for breaches of confidentiality and unauthorized disclosure of personal information requires ethical guidelines and standards of practice. The American Medical Association (AMA) code of ethics for physicians outlines several security measures if a breach occurs: Report to the affected individual quickly with a description of how it occurred and identify what specific information was leaked, the potential consequences of the breach, and the steps taken toward correcting the issue (Sade, 2010).

Preventive Measures and the EHR

Health care providers face challenges not only in keeping data private and secure, but also in determining who ultimately carries the responsibility for infractions against the security of that data. The degree of health care providers' responsibility will lie in their level of involvement with the system's security and integrity (Sade, 2010). Because of the varied and far-reaching implications of an EHR breach, such an error should be considered separately from a clinical error (Sade, 2010). Such a breach also changes what might constitute breaking bad news to a patient and family. This demonstrates that clinicians and patients/families must be further educated on the wide range of potential problems with the EHR to understand and discuss it in a meaningful way (Satkoske & Parker, 2010).

The following are preventive measures health care providers need to embrace to protect patient-related health:

- Monitoring protocols to prevent any unauthorized use of patient-related data

- Proper security measures identified and maintained by the institution

- Clinician understanding of the immediate and long-term implications of charting in the EHR

Nursing for the Future

The primary commitment of the nurse is to the patient, family, and community (American Nurses Association, 2001). To meet this commitment in the future, however, nurses need to be prepared with the skill sets necessary to understand the policies that impact the financing and delivery of health care for every patient, regardless of setting. Importantly, they will have to use not only their knowledge base but also their voices to address the cost and health-related inequities they face in day-to-day clinical interactions with patients.

In addition, "providers must be knowledgeable and up-to-date on the latest scientific evidence so that they can readily use the information to communicate 'what works and what doesn't' and provide evaluative advice to patients" (Ulrich & Grady, 2009; Veatch, 2009). In addition to evidence-based practice and ethical care, the World Health Organization (2005) identifies five complementary core competencies that will be essential to quality patient care throughout the 21st century and beyond.

World Health Organization Five Complementary Core Competencies for Quality Patient Care

1. Patient-centered care

2. Partnering with patients and other provider disciplines to communicate best practices

3. Quality improvement methodology

4. Informatics and communication technology

5. Systems thinking (or developing a public health perspective)

For example, the Affordable Care Act (ACA) was signed into law by President Obama in March 2010 with some health care reforms taking effect immediately and the majority being implemented through 2014. Many nurse leaders were initially involved in these discussions. Several important aspects of this bill are key for nursing care of patients in the future, such as embracing a patient-centered, systems-thinking approach. First, it provides basic coverage for millions of uninsured individuals in the United States. Secondly, it addresses some of the concerns associated with medical errors by fully implementing EHRs, thereby providing more efficient communication about patients' needs. Finally, "medical homes" will be established for children and adults with chronic illnesses (see Table 1.2).

Undoubtedly, nurses will continue to care for patients with complex health-related problems within a constrained economic environment and will continually be tested to work more efficiently and effectively to protect patients amidst the everyday ethical issues they encounter. Nurses will need to be armed with a host of interdisciplinary skills encompassing knowledge in areas such as biology, ethics, genetics and genomics, health policy, fiscal and economic policy, and communication sciences to care for patients in need of nursing advocacy in ways we have yet to fully recognize.

Benefits of the Affordable Care Act (ACA)

- Increased accountability and reform of abuses by insurance companies.
- Increased coverage for children; a ban on the denial of their coverage for pre-existing conditions.
- Termination of lifetime limits and annual limits on care.
- Permission for young adults (less than 26 years) to remain on their parents' health care insurance, unless they have employer-provided insurance of their own.
- Extension of the Medicare trust fund for 12 years.
- Increased payments for rural health care providers and incentives to grow the primary care workforce.
- Measures to decrease health care disparities.
- Deductions in the cost of brand name and generic drugs for Medicare recipients by elimination of the Medicare doughnut hole (Kocher, Emanuel, & DeParle, 2010).
- Transitional care for seniors (to keep them in their own homes and out of hospitals).

Conclusion

The future is always uncertain. What is clear, however, is that nursing's expertise is, and will remain, a valuable and critical component of the health care sector. In this chapter, we highlighted several challenging areas for nursing care in the future: an aging and chronically ill population, technological advancements, and health care reform initiatives—including the electronic health record (EHR). It seems plausible that an aging and chronically ill population will require new and innovative models of transitional care to meet their health care goals. In addition, new and improved patient-provider shared decision-making models promoting the involvement of patients and their families in key health-related decisions are an essential component of ethical care. Health care reform is a step forward—and in part, may not only address the rising costs of health care in terms of economics but also reduce the disparities in health outcomes for those individuals with limited or no health care coverage. Therefore, we have outlined several key components of the Affordable Care Act that nurses should be familiar with, as policy informs bedside practices and overall quality of care delivery. It is also true that difficult ethical questions and conversations surrounding end of life, palliative care, surrogate decision-making, and advance directives will need to take place. Finally, as outlined by the World Health Organization (2005), possessing interdisciplinary competencies such as systems thinking, informatics, and communication technology coupled with instruction in the humanities and basic sciences will be paramount. Nurses will need all of these skills as they continue to address the complex ethical issues at the bedside that are inevitable in future patient-provider relationships and the delivery of quality, cost-effective care.

Talk About It!

- How does an aging population affect your work today? How will it affect you in the next 5 years? Ten years? Talk to your colleagues about the impact caring for the elderly population will have in your clinical practice and additional safeguards that may be needed.

- What is the impact of the aging population on health care policy?

- Are you prepared to have an honest end-of-life dialogue with your patients? How can you start these discussions with patients at all stages of the lifespan? What role should families play in these discussions? What end-of-life communication skills do you need?

- What impact do you think the electronic health record will have on your patients' privacy and confidentiality? What can you do to maximize the protection of your patients' medical information?

References

Administration on Aging (AoA). (2011). *Aging statistics.* Retrieved from http://www.aoa.gov/AoARoot/Aging_Statistics/index.aspx

American Association of Colleges of Nursing (AACN). (2011). *Nursing shortage fact sheet.* Retrieved from http://www.aacn.nche.edu/media/FactSheets/NursingShortage.htm

American Nurses Association. (2001). *Code of ethics for nurses with interpretive statements.* Washington, DC: American Nurses Publishing. Retrieved from http://www.nursingworld.org/MainMenuCategories/ThePracticeofProfessionalNursing/EthicsStandards/CodeofEthics/

Associated Press. (2010). *1 in 7 Medicare patients harmed during hospital stay: 44 percent of the adverse events were preventable, government report says.* Retrieved from http://www.msnbc.msn.com/id/40220925/ns/health-health_care/

Blumenthal, D., & Tavenner, M. (2010). The "meaningful use" regulation for electronic health record. New England Journal of Medicine, *363*(6), 501-504.

Brazil, K., Kassalainen, S., Plorg, J., Marshall, D. (2010). Moral distress experienced by healthcare professionals who provide home-based palliative care. *Social Science and Medicine, 71*(9), 1687-91.

Catlin, A., Armigo, C., Volat, D., Vale, E., Hadley, M. A., Gong, W., & Anderson, K. (2008). Conscientious objection: A potential neonatal nursing response to care orders that cause suffering at the end of life? Study of a concept. *Neonatal Network, 27*(2), 101-108.

CBS News. (2010). The cost of dying. Retrieved from http://www.cbsnews.com/stories/2009/11/19/60minutes/main5711689.shtml

Centers for Disease Control and Prevention and The Merck Company Foundation. (2007). *The state of aging and health in America.* Whitehouse Station, NJ: The Merck Company Foundation. Retrieved from www.cdc.gov/aging

Centers for Medicare & Medicaid Services (CMS). (2011). *Definition of electronic health record.* Retrieved from http://www.cms.gov/EHealthRecords/

Federal Interagency Forum on Aging-Related Statistics. (2010). *Older Americans 2010: Key indicators of well-being.* Washington, DC: U.S. Government Printing Office.

Ferrell, B. (2006). Understanding the moral distress of nurses witnessing medically futile care. *Oncology Nursing Forum, 33*(5), 922-30.

Gabrielle, S., Jackson, J., & Mannix, J. (2008). Older women nurses: Health, aging concerns, and self-care strategies. *Journal of Advanced Nursing, 61*(3), 316-325.

Gavrin, J. (2007). Ethical considerations at end of life in the ICU. *Critical Care Medicine, 35*(Suppl.), S85-S94.

Gillick, M. R. (2009). Potential burdens of low-tech interventions near the end of life. *Journal of Pain and Symptom Management, 37*(3), 429-432.

Hinds, P. S., Oakes, L., Furman, W., Quargnenti, A., Olson, M. S., Foppiano, P., & Srivastava, D. K. (2001). End-of-life decision making by adolescents, parents, and health care providers in pediatric oncology: Research to evidence-based practice guidelines. *Cancer Nursing, 24*(2), 122-34.

Ivashkov, Y., & Van Norman, G. A. (2009). Informed consent and the ethical management of the older patient. *Anesthesiology Clinics, 27*(3), 569-580.

Jairath, N., Ulrich, C. M., & Ley, C. (2005). Ethical considerations in the recruitment of research subjects from hospitalized, cardiovascular patient populations. *Journal of Cardiovascular Nursing, 20*(1), 56-61.

Jones, J. M. (2010). *Nurses top honesty and ethics for 11th year in a row.* Retrieved from http://www.gallup.com/poll/145043/Nurses-Top-Honesty-Ethics-List-11-Year.aspx

Kleyman, P. (2009, January 25). Advocates for ethic elders look beyond inaugural euphoria. *New America media.* Retrieved from http://news.newamericamedia.org/news/view_article.html?article_id=5578da8651e7a1e83d60514e88a3f7c7

Kocher, R., Emanuel, E. J., & DeParle, N. M. (2010). The affordable care act and the future of clinical medicine: The opportunities and challenges. *Annals of Internal Medicine, 153*(8), 536-539.

Kriecbergs, U., Valdimarsdottir, U., Onelov, E., Henter, J., & Steineck, G. (2004). Anxiety and depression in parents 4-9 years after the loss of a child owing to a malignancy: A population-based follow-up. *Psychological Medicine, 34*(8), 1431-1441.

Landefeld, C.S. (2003). Training in the care of older adults. *Journal of General Internal Medicine, 18*(9), 770-771.

Piers, R., Van den Eynde, M., Stelman, E., Vlerick, P., Benoit, D., Van den Noortgate (2011). End of life of the geriatric patient and nurses' moral distress. *Journal of the American Medical Directors Association.* In press ahead of print. DOI: 10.1016/j.jamda.2010.12.014

Rushton, C. (2006). Defining and addressing moral distress: Tools for critical care nursing leaders. *AACN Advances in Critical Care, 17*(2), 161-8.

Sade, R. M. (2010). Breaches of health information: Are electronic records different from paper records? *The Journal of Clinical Ethics, 21*(1), 39-41.

Satkoske, V. B., & Parker, L. S. (2010). Practicing preventive ethics, protecting patients: Challenges of the electronic health record. *The Journal of Clinical Ethics, 21*(1), 36-38.

Sittig, D. F., & Singh, H. (2011). Legal, ethical, and financial dilemmas in electronic health record adoption and use. *Pediatrics, 127,* e1042-e1048.

Solomon, M. Z., Sellers, D. E., Heller, K. S., Dokken, D. L., Levetown, M., Rushton, C., … Fleischman, A. R. (2005). New and lingering controversies in pediatric end-of-life care. *Pediatrics, 116*(4), 872–883.

Thai, J. N. (2010, March 23). *How the 2009-2010 recession is impacting older minorities in the US.* Retrieved from: http://www.globalaging.org/elderrights/us/2010/usminorities.pdf

Ulrich, C., & Grady, C. (2009). Doing "good" with limited resources: Is it good enough in the provision of quality clinical care? *Clinical Scholars Review, 2*(1), 5-7.

Veatch, R. M. (2009). *Patient, heal thyself: How the new medicine puts the patient in charge.* New York: Oxford University Press.

Wolfe, J., Grier, H., Klar, N., Levin, S. B., Ellenbogen, J. M., Salem-Schatz, S., Emanuel, E. J., & Weeks, J. C. (2000). Symptoms and suffering at the end of life in children with cancer. *The New England Journal of Medicine, 342*(5), 326-333.

World Health Organization (WHO). (2005). *Preparing a health care workforce for the 21st century: The challenge of chronic conditions.* Retrieved from: http://www.who.int/chp/knowledge/publications/workforce_report.pdf

ETHICAL DECISION-MAKING: A FRAMEWORK FOR UNDERSTANDING AND RESOLVING MENTAL HEALTH DILEMMAS

2

–Marna S. Barrett, PhD
Clinical Associate Professor of Psychology in Psychiatry
University of Pennsylvania Perelman School of Medicine

Think About It!

- Ethical dilemmas are inherently troublesome, primarily because they involve at least two competing yet equally "right" choices rather than a right versus wrong choice.

- Distinct from other branches of medicine, psychiatry raises unique challenges for ethical decision-making. Only in mental health are we asked to determine a person's competence, restrict a person's right to self-determination, participate in legal decisions about a person's culpability, and engage with society in a reciprocal relationship of influence.

- Ethical principles such as autonomy, beneficence, nonmaleficence, fidelity, justice, and empathy are ideals to which we strive. Although useful for understanding the complexities of a dilemma, they are not sufficient for problem resolution.

- A framework for ethical decision-making is imperative for developing a consistent and effective personal standard for resolving ethical dilemmas. Key elements of such a framework include identifying and clarifying the issue, determining whether the situation is a "right versus wrong" or a "right versus right" dilemma, evaluating the principles involved, creating a "trilemma," weighing benefits and burdens, consulting, considering possible outcomes, making document decisions, and reviewing and reflecting on the process.

Ethical dilemmas are among the most difficult struggles we face. Whether in our professional or personal lives, we are confronted with decisions about what is right, fair, kind, and just. Within medicine, ethical dilemmas are more pronounced because of competing concerns such as benefit versus harm, the rights of individuals versus the rights of others, patient competency, patient versus hospital obligations, or truth versus kindness. In all ways, we are encouraged by our profession to strive toward the ideals of "compassion and respect for the inherent dignity, worth, and uniqueness of every individual" (American Nurses Association (ANA, 2001, para. 16). A formal code of ethics is what enables professionals to make clear to society the ethical obligations and duties that can be expected from us.

Being ethical, however, involves more than simply adhering to a professional code of ethics; it requires the infusion of personal virtues and ideals. For example, two nurses can follow the same mandate to respect others, yet someone who holds the personal ideal of autonomy and self-determination is likely to uphold a patient's ideas, beliefs, and decisions, even if these are in conflict with the opinion of a colleague. Differing personal values help explain why conflict so frequently arises between two ethically sound individuals.

Although the *Code of Ethics for Nurses* (ANA, 2001) guides and directs our thinking about ethical behavior, it provides little help in determining a course of action we should take when faced with a specific dilemma. In fact, what makes an ethical dilemma a dilemma is that two possible solutions exist, neither of which seems fully acceptable. Without some type of framework to guide the decision-making process, we are left to our own feelings, beliefs, hunches, and best bets about the "right" action.

In this chapter, I first discuss the general nature of decision-making, how decision-making differs in the context of a moral dilemma, and why a model of moral decision-making specific to mental health issues is needed. I then present the organizing principles of ethics and how they can be used to inform decisions. I then cover five models or frameworks for decision-making that are useful in addressing and resolving ethical dilemmas across contexts or situations. I end with a case presentation using the practice-based model for decision-making, one that I have found to be comprehensive, easy to use, and widely applicable to ethical issues in mental health.

Decision-Making

When faced with any decision, we generally follow three steps.

1. We identify the various alternatives for action. So, if I'm unhappy in my current position, I might consider quitting, moving to another hospital floor or unit, working on a different shift, or returning to school.

2. After all possibilities are identified, we review the potential outcome of each. For example, quitting might present financial difficulties, working a different shift might not be feasible given childcare responsibilities, and moving to another floor would mean switching from geriatrics to medical/surgical.

3. Having considered all the possibilities and outcomes, we make a choice between the alternatives based on personal values and preferences. For example, although I am unhappy in my current position, I value the time with my children and believe that I am especially gifted in working with older patients. Therefore, I decide to remain where I am and look for ways to change the environment so that I feel happier.

But how does decision-making related to moral or ethical issues differ? First, the dilemmas or uncertainties concern moral issues and, as such, are inherently personal. Although societies typically hold to a set of moral values, such as honesty, respect, kindness, fairness, and freedom, the range of values and the importance given to a particular value are unique to each individual. Whereas some people value honesty above all else, others value tolerance and appreciation of differences; and still others value faith, integrity, personal happiness, or hard work. Because morals influence our behavior, they are considered personal characteristics and thus carry emotional weight. When a dilemma arises that involves moral issues, we are faced not only with choosing among various alternatives for action but also with the emotion-laden values associated with any choice. In fact, the need for rationality (or reduction of emotion) in resolving ethical deliberations is the second factor unique to ethical decision-making.

Let's re-examine the dilemma about work (presented earlier) with the knowledge that my unhappiness is primarily related to conflict with my supervisor. Although I am someone who is deeply proud of my work and feels a strong commitment to the people and hospital where I work, I respect authority and find it hard to confront my supervisor. With this information selecting a course of action becomes more complicated. Quitting my job would risk financial hardship and create a tension between my values of respect for authority and commitment to others. Considering a change in shift could create a conflict between my need for happiness and my commitment to fellow employees and to my children. However, a move to another floor in the hospital would allow me to maintain my values and meet the needs of my family. Thus, situations that involve moral and ethical concerns invoke such emotional connections to the issue that rationality and rigor in making any decision are warranted.

Mental health issues complicate the picture even more. Unlike any other aspect of medicine, psychiatry has unique moral and ethical issues (Fulford & Hope, 1994; Radden, 2002). In no other branch of medicine are assessments of the competency of patients to make decisions about their care required. Medical philosophers such as Thomas Szasz (1959) have argued that restricting a person's right to self-determination is worse than slavery. Yet psychiatrists are typically asked to make such decisions so that other medical specialists can proceed with a particular course of action.

Mental health disciplines are also unique in that they play a role in legal issues—competency to stand trial, determination of sanity, or custody issues. Other than expert testimony, discussions of an individual's physical or medical health have little place in the courtroom and are not influential in determining legal outcomes. Mental health problems, in contrast, frequently influence the courts in terms of sentencing, guardianship, or responsibility for action.

Case Study 2.1

Jim, a 65-year-old white man with beginning dementia, was hospitalized with diverticulitis. He was operated on and had an unremarkable recovery. As part of his discharge planning, he was to be given Oxycontin for pain. Jim did not think there would be much pain and didn't want to take medication for fear that he would become dependent. Jim had recently seen a television show about addiction to painkillers and feared it might happen to him, since there was substance abuse in his family. Jim refused the prescription for Oxycontin and was told that he could not be discharged without it. The more the nurse tried to get Jim to accept the prescription (whether or not he actually took the medication), the angrier and more suspicious he became about the reasons for the medication.

This case presents several ethical challenges. For instance, should the nurse continue to deny discharge to Jim unless he accepts the prescription, or should the policy be waived? Although discharge planning is routinely handled by the nurse, should Jim's doctor be notified of the situation and asked to override the order for pain medication? Given Jim's problems with reasoning (i.e., beginning dementia), it might be useful to spend a few minutes educating him about the appropriate and safe use of pain medication. However, what should be done if he still refuses the prescription?

Additionally, a reciprocal relationship of influence exists between society and mental health. The Diagnostic and Statistical Manual of Mental Disorders (DSM-IV), published by the American Psychiatric Association (2000), offers a nosology for mental health disorders that determines the standard criteria by which behaviors are considered abnormal. By establishing such criteria, psychiatry influences what behavior is seen as problematic, justifies the need for treatment, and affects third-party payment. Secondary effects of behavioral labeling are social stigma, forced treatment, isolation, and marginalization.

A recent example of the reciprocal influence with society is the diagnosis of Asperger's syndrome. Although considered a part of the autism spectrum disorders, Asperger's syndrome was treated as a separate diagnosis in the DSM-IV because of the distinct symptomatic picture. This distinction resulted in greater awareness of the disorder, improved funding for research, and reduced stigma (Hamilton, 2010). However, in considering revisions for the new DSM-5, researchers have suggested that Asperger's syndrome be moved back under the rubric of autism spectrum disorders, because the basic difficulties with social engagement and language development are the same (Macintosh & Dissanayake, 2004). Not surprisingly, this suggestion has been met with considerable resistance and public outcry. Although many believe that the services available to individuals with Asperger's syndrome would increase, the fear is that such a move would damage the considerable progress made in terms of reduced stigma and social acceptance for this disorder (Parenting Aspergers, 2010).

Ethical decision-making is, therefore, the attempt to decide between at least two competing courses of action that is complicated by personal values, strong emotions, and unclear guidelines. When occurring in the context of mental health, ethical decision-making is further complicated by the social, personal, legal, and organizational filters through which the situation must be examined. For these reasons, a framework to guide and inform ethical decision-making is crucial.

Ethical Principles

Ethical principles are the standards that guide and promote the values held by a society, organization, or individual in determining what is right or wrong. Having their roots in ancient Greek philosophy, these principles are fundamental to Western bioethics (Beauchamp, 1999; Beauchamp & Childress, 2001) and form the basis for professional codes of ethics (Bloch & Pargiter, 1999).

- **Autonomy** refers to individuals' rights to make choices about the nature and direction of their life without interference from others. Respect for autonomy means that we recognize and appreciate an individual's perspective and capacities to hold certain views, make certain choices, and take action based on personal values, beliefs, and ideas.

- **Beneficence** is essentially seeing to the welfare of others. In medicine it requires us to act in ways that benefit others or are in their best interest. For example, patients benefit when we show mercy, kindness, or charity to them by alleviating their pain and suffering. Beneficence can also extend to aid we give in finding financial assistance or helping patients to gain access to health care.

- Somewhat in concert with beneficence, the principle of **nonmaleficence** requires action that does not bring harm to or hurt others. The balance between nonmaleficence and beneficence is one of the most common dilemmas within medicine, because most interventions or treatments involve the weighing of benefits versus risks.

- **Fidelity** refers to the act of faithfulness or loyalty. It is the trustworthiness people show in meeting their duties and obligations. Within medicine, fidelity also encompasses the trust patients place in us, the reliability and integrity of our treatments, and the manner in which these treatments are administered. Fidelity is of such importance that some have argued it is the foundation upon which all other ethical imperatives depend (Radden & Sadler, 2010).

- **Justice** can represent two types of behavior. Equal justice means treating all people the same without regard to any personal characteristic or behavior. Fairness refers to actions in which equal distributions of benefits, costs, and risks are made between individuals. For example, is a transplant list just in how it prioritizes individuals? Is it fair that someone of wealth can purchase a needed organ when others of lesser means are unable to do so?

- Although not always discussed as one of the fundamental ethical principles, **empathy** is a principle of behavior valued in medicine. Defined as the capacity to recognize and share the experience of others, empathy demonstrates an understanding of people and identification with their feelings that has been shown to affect outcome.

Case Study 2.2

Lisa, a critical-care nurse, is caring for Rochelle, a 73-year-old woman suffering from diabetes and multiple internal injuries following a serious motor vehicle accident. Although Rochelle had expressed to her husband and several friends a desire to not live in a situation as she was currently, her husband was persuaded by the children to do everything possible to sustain her life. Rochelle's husband has privately expressed to you his concern that her wishes are not being followed but feels he cannot disregard the wishes of their children.

What ethical dilemmas are raised in this case example? One challenge is whether or not Lisa should tell the doctors about Rochelle's stated desires for limited life support, since it is hearsay from her husband. Should Lisa discuss the situation with Rochelle's children? Should Rochelle's treatment be altered? Each of these dilemmas involves competing ethical principles. For example, underlying the decision to discuss Rochelle's desires with her doctors are the principles of beneficence (benefit to Rochelle by making her wishes known), fidelity (duty to disclose known information), and nonmaleficence (don't harm Rochelle by giving her treatment she would not want). However, in regard to any decision to alter treatment, the principle of beneficence (do what is in her best interest) may conflict with the principle of nonmaleficence (do her no harm). What other conflicts do you see between ethical principles?

Ethical principles are ideals to which we aspire and encourage us to act in ways that better us as individuals and as a part of society. They provide a level of organization to our thinking about what is moral or right and help inform ethical decisions (Beauchamp & Childress, 2001). In fact, the reason ethical situations are so challenging is precisely because these principles underlie our thinking, and individuals differ in what is valued. However, it should also be recognized that ethical standards and ideals are not obligations. We have no responsibility to adhere to them, and they should not form the basis for imposing sanctions. That said, let's now examine the ways these principles can inform our decisions.

Case Study 2.3

Betty is a 45-year-old Caucasian female with bipolar disorder, type II, who works as a nurse practitioner for Tisdale Internal Medicine. Her mood state has remained relatively stable for the past 15 years, with brief periods of moderately severe depression followed by mild hypomanic episodes. Six months ago, Betty suffered the loss of her mother, with whom she had a close relationship. She seemed to handle the loss well, but over the past month has become increasingly irritable, interrupting conversations and "talking over" others. She is currently full of energy, has several new ideas for improving office functioning, and feels the changes should be made immediately. Her demand for change has created tension among the staff, and patients have complained about her abrupt and somewhat dismissive behavior. Her boss, Dr. Mitchell, is aware of her recent loss, as well as her chronic mental health problems.

Dr. Mitchell is faced with the dilemma of determining how best to respond to Betty's behavior. Should Dr. Mitchell talk with Betty about her behavior, or should he intervene with staff? If he talks with Betty, what does he do if she refuses to acknowledge her behavior as problematic? How much of her history can be shared with the staff? To what extent does confidentiality restrict his range of responses? Consider these questions as we review several approaches to ethical dilemmas in the following section.

Ethics Principles Inform Decisions

Though meant to inspire us, ethical principles, such as those listed previously, also provide a basis for our thinking about ethical decisions. For example, the decision about how much to tell people prior to a surgical procedure, vaccination, or research participation (that is, informed consent) is grounded in the principles of autonomy, beneficence, nonmaleficence, justice, and empathy. Since the time of Aristotle and Plato, philosophers have argued about various ways to approach ethical situations that most benefit society. For example, from an Aristotelian perspective, society benefits when we recognize and further the goals we share in common, yet maintain respect for and value the freedom of individuals to pursue their own goals. Referred to as the fairness or justice approach, decisions are based on a determination of which action treats people most fairly.

Expanding this idea a bit further, the common good approach asks us to consider which action contributes most to the quality of life for the people involved. For example, of the number of ways to address the situation with Betty (Case Study 2.3), a common good approach would suggest that Dr. Mitchell talk with Betty about the effect her behavior has had on the office and encourage her to take time off and seek treatment.

A second major approach to ethical dilemmas is the act utilitarian or ends-based model. Utilitarian thinking requires consideration of which action brings the most benefit to the most people and incurs the least harm. Immanuel Kant was the main proponent of this approach and argued that in aspiring to higher principles, we need to consider our duties to others as well as to ourselves. If our motives are moral, then the outcome is considered moral and right. Applying this approach to the situation with Betty, Dr. Mitchell might decide to intervene more directly because of concerns about his patients as well as the staff. He could talk with Betty about her behavior and determine whether she needed to get treatment, if she was not already doing so. Although Dr. Mitchell values autonomy, in trying to balance the greatest benefit with the least harm he decides to override Betty's dismissal of the problems and calls her family.

A slightly different perspective to the ends-based model is referred to as rule utilitarianism. From this perspective, decisions are based on how much good is done by a particular action in regard to a rule or law. The premise is that the rules of society are in place to maintain order and are therefore to be respected and valued. For example, euthanasia, the ending of life to relieve pain and suffering, is legally wrong in this country. In deciding whether or not to continue life support of a comatose patient, a person following rule utilitarianism would consider how much society would benefit if life support were removed against the law.

A third major approach to ethical decision-making is rule-based or deontological thinking. This approach requires that we consider an action based on whether or not we would be comfortable with our action becoming law. In other words, the morality or ethic of an action is judged not on consequences, but on the principles that underlie the action. For example, in resolving the dilemma with Betty, Dr. Mitchell would determine a course of action consistent with his morals and values and one with which he would be comfortable as a standard for action.

Focusing more on individual character, the virtue-based approach to ethical decision-making encourages us to act in ways that are consistent with the person we want to be. Rather than focusing on the results of any action, virtue-based ethics focuses on becoming a person of good character. If Dr. Mitchell, in Case Study 2.3, held to a virtue-based approach, he might ask, "What kind of person should I be?" or "What action will promote the development of high moral character in me and my community?" or "If I take this action, will I become more like the person I want to be?"

The fifth major approach to ethical dilemmas is based on the principle of care (that is, the golden rule). Care-based thinking demands that we act in ways consistent with how we would want others to act toward us. This perspective considers inequalities in relationships, and priority is given to humane treatment that upholds the respect we all deserve as human beings. Applying this approach to the ongoing example of Betty, Dr. Mitchell would likely seek to understand how he would feel if he were Betty and base his decision for action on this understanding. Therefore, he might decide to talk with Betty about her behavior, help her to appreciate the negative effects brought on by the behavior, and together determine a course of action.

Why Are Ethical Decisions So Difficult?

Given the usefulness of ethical principles in informing decision-making strategies, why do we struggle so with these issues? Rushworth Kidder, in his book *How Good People Make Tough Choices* (1995), has articulated a simple yet poignant answer—most ethical dilemmas are not struggles of right versus wrong, but right versus right. Most of us have a fairly clear sense of what is right and wrong. Lying, cheating, and stealing are wrong. Respecting others, telling the truth, and being kind are right. However, at times we struggle with even these issues. For example, should you tell a patient about the availability of less invasive procedures when the physician they have seen always recommends surgery? Should Dr. Mitchell disclose his concerns about Betty to her family?

Despite such questions, most ethical dilemmas leave us unsure about a particular course of action precisely because they involve two competing "right" choices. For example, upholding patient confidentiality is right. However, breaking that confidentiality if it is for the protection of others (for example, HIV status, child abuse) is equally right. If you break confidentiality, the patient might no longer trust you and the therapeutic relationship will likely be damaged. If you don't break confidentiality, however, others might be hurt. Unfortunately, few clear legal mandates for taking a particular course of action exist, and our professional codes of ethics offer little in the way of specific guidelines for resolving dilemmas.

Four Paradigms Underlying Right Versus Right Dilemmas

1. Truth versus loyalty
2. Individual versus community
3. Short-Term versus long-term goals
4. Justice versus mercy

One way to begin to understand why "right versus right" dilemmas are so problematic is to recognize that often underlying these issues are competing moral paradigms. For example, being truthful is right and being loyal is equally right. Consider a scenario in which you've become aware that your agency is billing Medicare for therapy sessions that are not conducted in person, but over the phone. Providing some sessions by phone is the only way the psychiatrist can offer immediate care to patients in need. The dilemma, however, is whether you should be truthful and disclose the practice to Medicare or appreciate the efforts of the psychiatrist to provide care and maintain loyalty to the physicians and agency.

Another paradigm often underlying ethical dilemmas is the tension between an action that benefits the individual versus one that benefits the community. In my work with patients having bipolar disorder, I often struggle with the decision about hospitalization. Do I respect the autonomy and self-direction of the individual to decide whether or not hospital support is needed to control the manic behavior, or do I restrict his or her autonomy in favor of beneficence and decide that hospitalization is necessary for the welfare of the patient and community? This scenario might also be viewed as a struggle between beneficence and nonmaleficence. That is, do I help or harm the patient by allowing continued interactions that increase the likelihood of arguments, fights, uncontrolled spending, or other high-risk behavior? Is there a way I can help the patient, respect autonomy, and reduce the risk of harm? These are the issues that cause us discomfort and often lead to disagreements with others.

A third competing moral paradigm is that of short-term versus long-term goals. In my own life, deciding whether I should spend a Sunday afternoon writing papers that would further my career (a long-term goal) or spend an enjoyable day with my family (a relatively short-term goal) is an almost routine struggle. In the previous scenario about Medicare, the dilemma of greatest discomfort for the nurse might not be truth versus loyalty, but the conflict between her immediate need for employment (that is, I might be fired if I disclose the billing practices) and her long-term feelings about personal character (that is, I am becoming a bad person if I stay quiet and do not disclose something unethical). This situation highlights another important issue in understanding ethical dilemmas in that one issue can often be complicated by multiple competing paradigms.

One final paradigm often presenting itself in ethical dilemmas is that of justice versus mercy. This struggle is frequently at the heart of many jury deliberations. For example, should someone with schizophrenia be held accountable for his or her actions if he or she chose not to take prescribed medication? Should the sentence be lessened simply because of the diagnosis? The justice versus mercy debate is also central to decisions about removing life support or assisting the death of a terminally ill patient. Providing needed medical care is right and fair, and showing mercy by allowing a person to die with dignity is equally right and fair.

Although these are just a few of the more frequently occurring competing moral paradigms, this discussion clarifies why ethical dilemmas are so difficult and why we often disagree with respected friends and colleagues when faced with such a situation. Unfortunately, knowing why ethical issues are problematic does not get us any closer to knowing how to resolve them. Although professional codes of ethics, laws, and our own moral compass provide some guidance, they do not help in resolving the majority of issues we face, particularly in the area of mental health. Not knowing how to act when confronted with the gray areas of ethics is one of the main reasons I began to explore models of decision-making used in philosophy and business, with the hope that these might be applicable to mental health dilemmas.

Models of Ethical Decision-Making

A number of frameworks are useful in guiding decision-making; however, five models seem particularly appropriate when facing mental health decisions. These include the standards-based model, the principles-based model, the virtues-based model, the moral reasoning-based model, and the practice-based model. As a way to better understand and appreciate the strengths and limitations of these approaches, presentation of each model will incorporate discussion of the model's relevance to Case Study 2.4.

Case Study 2.4

Mr. Stevens is a 66-year-old divorced Caucasian man living alone. He has three grown children who live outside the state. Until 2 years ago, Mr. Stevens worked as a high school English teacher at a private school where he had been employed for 35 years. He took early retirement because of ill health and recently underwent cardiac bypass surgery for several blocked arteries. His rehabilitation following surgery went well, although he developed a severe depression during his stay in the rehabilitation facility. He has few friends and now is even more withdrawn, remaining isolated in his apartment watching TV. His financial situation has worsened, because he has been unable to find part-time employment and has little in savings. At a recent visit to his cardiologist, he mentioned to the nurse practitioner, Sophia, that he does not like taking "so many pills" and sometimes misses a dose. In passing, he mentioned that he would be better off if he had another heart attack and died. When Sophia suggested he speak with a mental health professional, Mr. Stevens said that he does not believe he is depressed, but just "worries some." He then stated quite adamantly that he did not want to burden his family with concerns of his situation.

Sophia is faced with several issues. Should she intervene with Mr. Stevens' family? Is treatment needed for Mr. Stevens? Is hospitalization warranted? Do social services need to be involved? How should Sophia handle questionable compliance with treatment? How might his recent surgery have influenced the depression, and does this impact her decision for intervention?

Standards-Based Model

The standards-based model for decision-making rests on the assumption that rules, laws, and policies provide the best basis for determining action. By holding to a standard set of rules for conduct, few situations are seen as ambiguous, and the only question to ask oneself is whether or not the situation warrants deviation from those rules. From this perspective, the first step in making a decision is to determine the primary dilemma. This might seem somewhat intuitive, but situations are often complicated by the presence of multiple clinical, social, legal, and ethical issues that often cloud our ability to appreciate the main dilemma to be addressed. For example, the case of Mr. Stevens involves issues related to suicidal thoughts, depression, the taking of medication, financial hardships, and lack of insight. However, the primary issue is whether or not to force some type of mental health treatment.

Standards-Based Model

1. Determine the primary dilemma.

2. What standards apply?

3. Determine a course of action.

4. Is there a reason to deviate?

Once we identify the key issue, the second step we take is to specify the standards that apply to the situation and determine whether we have reason to deviate. In Mr. Steven's case, the standard rule of care would be to arrange for a mental health appointment and follow up with him regarding compliance. Having determined the course of action, we can now ask if we have any reason to deviate from this standard. At this point, the model often fails us. For example, how severe does Mr. Stevens' depression have to be before we take a different action? Is his social isolation and firm decision not to inform his family enough to warrant deviation? Do we need to consider his denial of depression? With these questions in mind, we can examine a second model.

Principles-Based Model

A principles-based approach to decision-making relies on the philosophical principles of autonomy, beneficence, nonmaleficence, justice, loyalty, and empathy to guide our ethical thinking. There are four major steps in a principles-based approach: clarify the dilemma, evaluate the situation, decide on a course of action, and act. As with the standards-based approach, one of the first steps in addressing any dilemma is determination of the primary issue. In the example of Mr. Stevens, the key dilemma is whether or not to force some type of mental health treatment.

Principles-Based Model

1. Clarify the dilemma.
2. Evaluate the ethical principles/factors involved.
3. Decide on a course of action.
4. Act.

Having identified the primary problem, the principles-based approach probes more deeply into the issue and requires consideration of the ethical principles and values involved. In the case of Mr. Stevens, the underlying principles are autonomy (respecting his right to make decisions about his care), beneficence (act to benefit him), loyalty (to Mr. Stevens), truthfulness (to Mr. Stevens' family), and empathy. Knowing which principles are involved can help us clarify the dilemma and better evaluate the factors involved. For example, Sophia, the nurse practitioner, might need to ask Mr. Stevens for more information about why he doesn't want his family involved and how he understands his "worries," to distinguish facts from beliefs and opinions. This information can also help in weighing the benefits and burdens of any particular course of action, such as whether Mr. Stevens should be started on medication, his family should be notified, or social services should be contacted. Because the principles-based approach focuses on ethical principles, deciding on a particular action involves prioritizing of principles, which might differ between individuals. For example, Mr. Stevens' cardiologist might hold beneficence as primary, whereas Sophia might regard autonomy as paramount, thereby leading to differing decisions for action. In this case, considering the worst case scenario and potential consequences of a specific choice might be helpful, although a decision still might not be reached. The inability to resolve dilemmas because of competing ethical priorities leaves us in no better position than before we examined the dilemma and is a significant limitation of the principles-based model.

Virtues-Based Model

The virtues-based model considers that our dispositions and habits enable us to act according to the highest potential of our character and on behalf of our values. In other words, the kind of person that I am and strive to be determines how I act. From this perspective, we ask two major questions in dealing with an ethical dilemma: Which of X, Y, or Z choices are most consistent with my values or virtues? What kind of person will I become if I take X, Y, or Z action? Recall that virtues encompass behaviors or characteristics such as autonomy, beneficence, empathy, fidelity, justice, and nonmaleficence. In regard to the situation with Mr. Stevens, Sophia would be encouraged to examine her personal values and determine which course of action is most consistent. If she prides herself on being an empathic person who respects individual rights, Sophia might be more inclined to arrange for treatment or hospitalization for Mr. Stevens than to involve outside agencies or his family. However, if she holds strongly to truthfulness and connection to others, Sophia might be more likely to alert Mr. Stevens' family to his condition and encourage Mr. Stevens to involve them in any discussions about treatment.

> ### Virtues-Based Model
>
> 1. What kind of person will I become if I take a particular course of action?
>
> 2. What course of action is most consistent with my virtues?
>
> 3. Act accordingly.

Either approach would be appropriate and "right," although vastly different outcomes are likely to result. Therefore, one of the major limitations of the virtues-based approach is that it relies on the virtues of each individual to determine a particular course of action. If the dilemma involves only a single person, the model can be useful. However, the greater number of people involved in the process, the more difficult it is to reach agreement, because everyone differs to a greater or lesser extent in the virtues to which they strive.

Moral Reasoning-Based Model

The moral reasoning-based approach to ethical dilemmas, proposed by Jones (1991), argues that individuals reason on a higher moral level when the perception of moral intensity increases. In other words, the extent to which an individual is immersed in the ethical dilemma, the perceived importance of the issue (that is, risk for harm, social consensus), the immediacy of action, and the degree of impact (amount of harm or benefit) all factor into the level of moral reasoning used in resolving a dilemma. Given that ethical decision-making requires considerable time and effort, Jones argues that we rely on lower levels of moral reasoning (for example, self-interests, social expectations) when an issue is less intense and higher order reasoning (for example, ethical principles, abstract thinking) when the perception of intensity is high. Stated more simply, when the stakes are high, we give greater thought in determining a course of action.

> ### Moral Reasoning-Based Model
>
> 1. Recognize the moral issue and determine that action is needed.
>
> 2. Determine level of involvement.
>   - Individual & situational variables
>   - Factors of opportunity
>
> 3. What is the effect of the decision on others?
>   - Impact an individual or group
>   - Likelihood of harm
>   - Closeness to the issue
>   - Agreement with social norms

- Immediacy of action
- Severity of impact

4. Act.

Relying on the moral reasoning-based model, how might Sophia approach the situation with Mr. Stevens? What level of moral intensity might she perceive? As with several of the models, we must first recognize that a situation involves a moral issue requiring us to act. The moral reasoning approach then asks that we determine our level of involvement in the dilemma by assessing individual and situational factors. For example, because the situation with Mr. Stevens involves issues related to his care, both Sophia and the cardiologist are likely to be involved in the decision-making. However, because Mr. Stevens disclosed his feelings to Sophia and she has a relationship with him, she is in a better position than the cardiologist to intervene. The next major step is to determine the effect of any decision on others. For example, although Mr. Stevens' family would be affected if the decision was made to contact them or pursue hospitalization, the main person affected by any decision is Mr. Stevens. Also involved in determining the effect of a decision is whether harm might come to Mr. Stevens as a result. Although physical harm is unlikely, Mr. Stevens could well suffer from forced treatment, unwanted interactions with his family, or challenges to his self-esteem. In regard to the issues, the need for treatment and potential for self-harm are important social concerns, and a decision to contact Mr. Stevens' family, refer him for treatment, or hospitalize him if at risk for suicide would be deemed by most of society as appropriate courses of action.

Two final considerations are whether the decision needs to be made immediately and the severity of its impact. The question of immediacy is fairly straightforward. Mr. Stevens does not report clear intent or plan for suicide and is functioning well, albeit with some limitation. So those involved have time to consider various options and to even meet with Mr. Stevens again. Despite these less immediate concerns, the decision does have fairly significant consequences for the doctor-patient relationship, relationships with family, Mr. Stevens' self-perception, and follow-through on treatment. So the moral intensity of the situation for Sophia is moderately high and requires more than consideration of her interests and desires or those of society. Although Sophia needs to give considerable thought before acting, she is still left to make a decision without much more guidance than consideration and prioritization of her ethical principles.

Practice-Based Model

Each of the models discussed so far is useful for guiding our understanding of ethical dilemmas and the issues involved, but none addresses the fact that most dilemmas involve tension between two competing "right" choices. Furthermore, none of the models is comprehensive enough to facilitate decision-making across a number of different situations or contexts. Because legal mandates, professional guidelines, and personal virtues provide only a modicum of direction when we are faced with an ethical dilemma, and any decision we make can be and often is scrutinized and challenged, we need to develop a model for ethical decision-making that is comprehensive, yet simple enough to allow a "standard for action" that we can routinely follow.

The practice-based model, developed from the work of Rushworth Kidder (1995), incorporates the key aspects of the standards, principles, virtues, and moral reasoning-based approaches into a simple frame-work based on the premise that most dilemmas are not moral issues of "right versus wrong," but rather "right versus right" dilemmas. In the dilemma confronted by Sophia, the practice-based approach would suggest that she first ask whether or not the situation involves a moral issue. Though this might seem rather superfluous, many dilemmas are primarily clinical or legal concerns rather than moral ones. For example, maintaining confidentiality in the therapeutic setting is a clinical mandate. However, if I have knowledge about child abuse or the potential for harm, I am legally mandated to break confidentiality and report the information—regardless of any ethical or moral concerns. In the case of Sophia and Mr. Stevens, the issue involves both ethical (for example, disclosure) and clinical concerns (compliance, treatment). Having clarified the ethical concerns, I can now address the appropriate issues.

Practice-Based Model

1. Recognize the moral issue.
2. Determine the individuals involved.
3. Gather the relevant facts.
4. Test for right versus wrong issues.
5. Test for right versus right paradigms.
6. Determine resolution principles involved.
7. Investigate "trilemma."
8. Weigh benefits & burdens.
9. Consult.
10. Consider dilemmas resulting from action.
11. Make the decision.
12. Formulate a justification for the decision.
13. Document.
14. Review & reflect.

From a moral reasoning or practice-based perspective, the next step would be consideration of the moral intensity of the dilemma. Who are the individuals involved? How immediately is a decision need-ed? What is the potential impact of this decision? As you might recall, we determined previously that So-phia's dilemma was moderately intense and, therefore, requires careful moral consideration. So, what are the relevant facts? Mr. Stevens is depressed, not functioning well, withdrawn from family and friends, and has passive suicidal thoughts. Sophia is the only person to whom this information is known. Sophia works for the cardiologist who recently operated on Mr. Stevens. Mr. Stevens does not appreciate the severity of his depression and has adamantly stated that he does not want his family informed.

Having identified the key players in the dilemma and the facts involved, we return to consideration of the moral and ethical concerns. Is the issue of disclosure a "right versus wrong" decision, or is it a "right versus right" dilemma? One quick test helpful in making this determination is what Kidder (1995) has referred to as the "front page" test. Stated more fully, I ask, "Would I be comfortable having my decision published on the front page of the paper?" Although some nurses might view disclosure as a clear-cut "wrong" decision, most would agree that the issue of disclosing Mr. Stevens' depression is not so straight-forward and encompasses competing "right" choices. But what are the "right" choices?

As discussed earlier in the chapter, four basic paradigms underlie "right versus right" dilemmas and all underscore the dilemma with Mr. Stevens. For example, Sophia wants to be truthful about Mr. Stevens' situation but also feels loyal to him and respects his right to privacy. Although the decision about disclosure primarily involves Mr. Stevens, Sophia must also consider the implications for Mr. Stevens' family and the cardiology practice. Mr. Stevens' short-term needs are for improved functioning and self-care. Equally important, however, are long-term goals of family support, health, and happiness. Finally, tension exists between justice and mercy. Although Sophia wants to be just and fair in getting Mr. Stevens whatever care he needs, she also feels merciful toward him and wants to respect his wishes.

Having gained a better understanding about the "right versus right" nature of her dilemma, Sophia can now reflect on the ethical principles she values and how these influence her thinking. Awareness of the underlying principles can also help Sophia in her discussions with the cardiologist, who might disagree with her about an appropriate action. From an ends-based approach, Sophia might decide to do whatever is necessary to get Mr. Stevens the treatment he needs for his depression. However, notifying Mr. Stevens' family against his will might not be a "rule" for action that Sophia would want adopted, and thus, she might consider how she would want to be treated if in the same situation. If she values an individual's right to self-determination, Sophia would likely seek ways to support Mr. Stevens' decision while also getting him the care he needs.

Sophia now has a clear perspective on the dilemma, its ethical underpinnings, and the issues with which she struggles in reaching a decision. At this point, she must consider a course for action. One of the most useful aspects of Kidder's approach to decision-making is the suggestion that, rather than focusing on the two-choice "dilemma," we instead focus on the "trilemma" in which multiple (at least three) possibilities for action are explored. Demanding that consideration be given to at least three options frees us from the "either or" mentality and allows us to be creative in developing strategies for resolution.

For example, rather than Sophia deciding between disclosure or nondisclosure of Mr. Stevens' depression to his family, she might decide to talk with Mr. Stevens about her concerns and educate him about depression. She could also discuss various ways to help his worry that would be agreeable to him (for example, increase his daily activity, encourage time with friends or family, arrange for him to attend a support group, give him referrals for therapy, consider medication). Sophia could also schedule an appointment for Mr. Stevens to talk with the cardiologist about his worries or arrange for him to meet with his primary physician, if he has a good relationship there. As this example illustrates, encouraging exploration of actions beyond the initial dilemma lessens the emotional intensity of the situation and fosters clearer perspective. Some of the most complicated decisions I have faced have been resolved in the most satisfying way solely because I pushed myself to develop at least three ways for action.

Reflective Practice

1. How would you prioritize the moral paradigms underlying Sophia's dilemma?

2. What ethical principles would guide your decision-making?

3. What other ways could Sophia's concerns about Mr. Stevens be addressed?

Having several strategies for dealing with Mr. Stevens' depression, Sophia must now make a decision. How does she decide? As with any decision, the benefits and costs of each decision must be considered. If Sophia decides to delay disclosure and arranges for Mr. Stevens to talk with his family doctor, how does she know that he will follow through? What if nothing comes of the meeting? What is her obligation to Mr. Stevens beyond the referral? In weighing the risks and benefits of any decision, I have found it extremely useful to consult with my colleagues. Not only does this give me fresh perspective on the situation, but in this age of unrestrained litigation, consultation allows the blame for any decision to be shared. This might sound rather harsh, but sharing the burden for a decision can be reassuring, provide me with professional support, and lend credence to my decision as a standard to which others agree (Hedges, 2007).

One last consideration before making the decision is to reflect on the potential consequences of the action. More specifically, considering whether additional dilemmas might arise as a result of the decision is often helpful. For example, Sophia does not know how Mr. Stevens' family will respond if she decides to contact them. What does she do if they are angry with Mr. Stevens for not notifying them sooner? What if they are not interested? If she decides to refer him to his primary physician, what does she do if Mr. Stevens does not keep the appointment? What if the physician doesn't recognize the severity of his depression? Giving thought to potential outcomes allows us to recognize possible shortcomings of a decision and to anticipate possible objections.

Adapting the Practice-Based Model

Don't let the number of steps in the model scare you. It is comprehensive but can be shortened to quickly address whatever dilemma arises. You will also find that after only a few applications of the model, the steps flow fairly naturally.

Having carefully considered all aspects of the dilemma, it is now time to make the decision. However, our work is not yet done. Given that few mandates for action exist and most dilemmas are in ethical gray areas, decisions such as these need to be documented and defended. By clearly articulating the steps taken in reaching the decision, alternatives for action considered, justifications for the decision, limitations of the decision, and consultations, the seriousness with which the action is considered is demonstrated. Such behavior will not necessarily prevent legal or professional sanctions should others disagree with the decision. However, delineating the care taken in reaching a decision and having a set model by which we approach ethical dilemmas allow us to act in ways that are consistent with who we are and who we want to become. Even without clear moral or legal guidelines for behavior, we can act in virtuous ways.

Finally, we need to review the decision-making process and reflect on the outcome of the decision after the situation has resolved. What aspects of the situation were overlooked? Were there issues we failed to consider? How could this be avoided in the future? Were we able to consider the situation objectively? Are there ways the model could be altered to better aid our decision-making? Such reflection allows us to develop an approach to decision-making that is malleable, relevant, and personal. For example, when I am confronted with an ethical dilemma, all too often the emotion of the situation is so compelling, I fail to take time to carefully think the situation through and instead quickly jump to a decision. Because of this tendency, my own model of decision-making starts with the admonishment to "STOP. Take a deep breath." Only a few seconds of stepping away from the issue allows me to more carefully address the pertinent aspects of the situation and make an informed decision.

Conclusion

Throughout this chapter we have discussed the ethical challenges faced by nurses and how such dilemmas can be resolved. Although a formal code of ethics delineates expectations for behavior, our personal virtues and ideals are what enable us to act ethically. However, two ethically sound individuals may disagree on a course of action precisely because their personal values differ. Reaching a decision about an ethical situation is further complicated because typically there are at least two competing, equally right choices rather than a right and wrong choice.

Ethical decision-making is particularly challenging in the field of psychiatry. Only in mental health does society influence diagnostic decisions and ask us to make judgments about competence, right to self-determination, and culpability. Thus, a framework for understanding and addressing mental health dilemmas is imperative if we are to have a standard of care for consistent and effective resolution. Building on four major models of decision-making, the practice-based approach to ethical decision-making incorporates the ethical principles of philosophy into the practical decision-making strategies of business. Key elements of such a framework include identification and clarification of the issue, distinction between a "right versus wrong" or "right versus right" dilemma, evaluation of the principles involved, creation of a "trilemma," weighing of benefits and burdens, consultation, and consideration of possible outcomes. Following a decision, it is critically important that we document the steps we took in making the decision and give time to review and reflect on the process.

I encourage you to use the principles, paradigms, and models discussed in this chapter to develop your own framework for ethical decision-making. Not all of these will be applicable to you, your specialty, or your work setting, but they can offer a foundation from which you can create a personal model for effectively confronting and dealing with ethical dilemmas.

Talk About It!

- Think about the last week you worked. What ethical situations did you face? Did any involve "right vs. wrong" decisions or "right vs. right" dilemmas? What was the resolution? How did you feel about the process and/or outcome? Share your explorations about this situation with a colleague or your team. Discuss the different reactions each of you had regarding the situation.

- Think about one particularly challenging ethical situation.

- Which ethical principles were involved?

    - What were the competing moral paradigms?

    - What courses of action were considered?

    - How might it have helped to apply one of the models discussed in this chapter?

    - In what ways would the models be less helpful?

    - Explore this situation with someone in your life who is nonjudgemental but is thoughtful of similar situations so that you can explore the situation with a "devil's advocate."

- Discuss this same situation with a trusted colleague to explore the ethical principles he or she values, what approach he or she would likely take, and what creative ideas for resolution he or she offers. In what ways do you agree or disagree?

References

American Nurses Association (ANA). (2001). *Code of ethics for nurses.* Retrieved from http://nursingworld.org.MainMenuCategories/EthicsStandards/CodeofEthicsforNurses/Code-of-Ethics.pdf

American Psychiatric Association. (2000). *Diagnostic and statistical manual of mental disorders: Text revision* (DSM-IV-TR; 4th ed.). Washington, DC: Author.

Beauchamp, T. L. (1999). The philosophical basis of psychiatric ethics. In S. Bloch, P. Chodoff, & S. A. Green (Eds.), *Psychiatric ethics* (3rd ed.; pp. 25-48). New York: Oxford University Press.

Beauchamp, T. L. & Childress, J. F. (2001). *Principles of biomedical ethics* (5th ed.; pp. 1-21). New York: Oxford University Press, Inc.

Bloch, S., & Pargiter, R. (1999). *Codes of ethics in psychiatry.* In S. Bloch, P. Chodoff, & S. A. Green (Eds.), Psychiatric ethics (3rd ed.; pp. 81-103). New York: Oxford University Press.

Fulford, K. W. M., & Hope, T. (1994). Psychiatric ethics: a bioethical ugly duckling? In R. Gillon & A. Lloyd (Eds.), *Principles of health care ethics* (pp. 681-695). New York : John Wiley & Sons, 1994.

Hamilton, J. (2010, February 10). *Asperger's officially placed inside autism spectrum* [Radio broadcast]. USA: National Public Radio.

Hedges, L. E. (2007). *Facing the challenge of liability in psychotherapy: Practicing defensively* (2nd ed.). Lanham, MD: Rowan and Littlefield Publication Group.

Jones, T. (1991). Ethical decision making by individuals in organizations: An issue-contingent model. *Academy of Management Review, 16*(2), 366-395.

Kidder, R. M . (1995). *How good people make tough choices: Resolving the dilemmas of ethical living.* New York: William Morrow.

Macintosh, K. E., & Dissanayake, C. (2004). The similarities and differences between autistic disorder and Asperger's disorder: A review of the empirical evidence. *Journal of Child Psychology and Psychiatry, 45*(3), 421-434.

Parenting Aspergers. (2010, April 7). Aspergers diagnosis and the DSM 5 proposed changes. *Parenting Aspergers Blog.* Retrieved from http://parentingaspergers.com/blog/other/aspergers-diagnosis-and-the-dsm-5-proposed-changes

Radden, J. (2002). Notes towards a professional ethics for psychiatry. *Australian and New Zealand Journal of Psychiatry, 36*(1), 52-59.

Radden, J., & Sadler, J. Z. (2010). *The Virtuous Psychiatrist.* New York: Oxford University Press, Inc.

Szasz, T. (1959). The myth of mental illness. *American Psychologist, 15*, 113-118.

FINDING A VOICE IN ETHICS: EVERYDAY ETHICAL BEHAVIOR IN NURSING

3

–Lucia D. Wocial, PhD, RN
Nurse Ethicist, Indiana University Health
Adjunct Assistant Professor, Indiana University School of Nursing

Think About It!

- Speaking up in ethically challenging situations is a skill that takes practice.
- Finding your voice to express your values is the right thing to do for your patients and for yourself.
- Ethically challenging situations can be found in the seemingly mundane activities of routine nursing care.
- Nurses must cultivate a sense of moral courage to uphold the trust the public has placed in them.

If doing the right thing were easy, no one would need to study ethics. In any given situation, nurses might find more than one right thing to do, and it might not be clear which right thing someone should do. Studying ethics in a formal way can assist nurses with developing knowledge of what the right thing to do is. Knowledge alone, however, does not help nurses develop the skills necessary to act in challenging situations. In addition, the focus in ethics on the big topics (for example, end-of-life care, transplants, and clinical research) fails to help nurses appreciate and practice the skills necessary to navigate the everyday circumstances that define ethical behavior.

Ethical competence depends on being able to detect ethically challenging situations and contemplate different courses of action—but most importantly, to take action. Arguably one of the most powerful actions is speaking, giving values a voice. This means that nurses must learn to use their voices to speak up and influence the course of events through careful, intentional communication. Competence in ethics demands first that nurses reflect on and articulate their everyday ethical concerns and not limit their understanding to ethical breakdowns and dilemmas. Genuine awareness of ethics unfolds in the concrete reality of what nurses live every day, not in the philosophical contemplation of right and wrong. Learning to apply ethics is a personal transformation that happens in the complex and ambiguous events of everyday nursing.

Nurses are consistently identified as the most trusted professional in Gallup polls. That trust demands that nurses take care of their patients. People look to nurses for support and see them as the person who can advocate on their behalf. People believe nurses will speak up for them even, and perhaps especially, in challenging situations. Nurses are expected to exercise moral courage and act on ethical principles and values to help others in difficult ethical situations, even when those nurses face personal risk by acting.

Exercising moral courage requires that nurses find a strong moral compass that guides them in situations where giving voice to their values matters most. Nurses might feel they are more adept at communication because they receive special training in therapeutic communication. However, speaking up in challenging situations requires more than training in therapeutic communication. This chapter identifies reasons why speaking up matters, explores the compelling evidence that nurses are falling short on this front, and offers strategies for developing the necessary skills to find your voice when it matters.

Finding a moral compass requires that you exercise your imagination and consider who you want to be as a nurse. More importantly, it depends on doing something, taking action. If all you plan to do is read this chapter, stop now. The challenge for readers of this chapter is to reflect on experiences in clinical practice and apply the lens of ethics, and thereby clarify the meaning of ethics in day-to-day clinical practice. Reflection is an opportunity to explore other perspectives that can shed light on the application of ethics to similar situations in the future.

Practice what you want to be, either by talking to others about it or doing real exercises that will help you imagine a positive outcome when you speak your values (Gentile, 2010). Speaking up is not just about what you say but how you say it. The first part of this chapter is about whether or not to do it. The second part is about how to do it. Start by considering and writing down your answers to these basic questions:

1. What defines me as a person?

2. Who do I wish to be?

3. What behaviors will exemplify this person?

4. Think of a time when you spoke up in defense of your values. Describe the situation. (What happened, what did you say, and how did you say it?)

Everyday Ethical Comportment

A recent Carnegie report on transforming nursing education devoted a significant amount of content to the development of everyday ethical comportment, or behavior (Benner, Sutphen, Leonard, & Day, 2010). The report discusses the importance of nurses learning to behave in an ethical manner in part because the true challenge to ethical comportment is not in the dramatic ethical dilemmas, but in the day-to-day conflicts nurses face, when doing the right thing is hard. Imagine you are the nurse in the case studies that follow. Then, write down your responses to the questions following those case studies before continuing in the chapter.

Case Study 3.1

You are caring for a patient who needs a central line placed. When the physician arrives to place the line at bedside, she asks for sterile gloves and drapes and begins cleaning the intended insertion site. When you ask her to wear a sterile gown, hat, and mask she refuses, stating she has no time for those details, and besides, it is a local procedure. You remind her that these measures are part of standard policy and procedure and part of an initiative to decrease blood stream infections in your institution. She responds by yelling at you and telling you to get out and send in a more helpful nurse. What is a right thing to do in this situation? What might pressure the nurse to take the path of least resistance and fail to do a right thing?

Case Study 3.2

You are a new nurse orienting to a nursing unit. One of your patients has an order for blood cultures. On previous days, you learned that when blood cultures are ordered, the policy is to draw two separate cultures from two different sites 20 minutes apart. The unit is busy, and your preceptor for the day states there is no time to do two separate draws. She tells you to draw two samples from the same site, 5 minutes apart, and chart that they were drawn according to policy. What is a right course of action for this new nurse? What are the consequences to the patient if the nurse fails to do a right thing?

Case Study 3.3

One of the patients in your care has MRSA and is in contact isolation, with signs clearly posted reminding people to wear protective gowns and gloves when entering the room. The patient has been in isolation for several days, and his spouse has been a daily visitor. When the patient's spouse arrives on the unit, she attempts to enter the patient's room without wearing a protective gown or gloves. When you stop her to remind her to put on the protective gear, she shouts at you. She says that you are mean and tells you that other nurses let her go in without the gown. If you continue to bother her, she says she will speak to the manager. What is a right thing to do in this situation? What are the consequences to the nurse if she fails to do a right thing?

These situations might seem trivial when compared with such weighty ethical questions such as whether treatment should be withdrawn or withheld. However, these day-to-day conflicts challenge a nurse to be true to the foundational values of nursing. There is no one right thing to do in any of these three case studies. The list of possible actions in any given scenario is endless. Doing a right thing is not easy for countless reasons, including fearing retaliation, wanting to fit in, and avoiding conflict. Yet failing to do a right thing in these situations can potentially result in harm to the patient. For nurses, knowing there is a right thing to do and failing to do it erode their integrity and self-respect. That inaction represents a failure to address the moral issue.

The complexity of managing these situations to achieve the best outcome for the patient demands high-level communication skills from nurses. Nurses have more to manage than meeting the patient's needs. They must take action to protect the patient, but must also choose what to do regarding the unprofessional behavior of a colleague or inappropriate behavior of a patient's family member.

In Case Study 3.1, the authority gradient issue between physicians and nurses is a barrier to challenging the physician's behavior and continuing to advocate on behalf of the patient. The authority gradient issue is also present in the second scenario, but it is more insidious because it is nurse on nurse and reinforces an attitude of "If everyone else is doing it, and they don't get caught, why should I do anything different?" Finally, in the last example, a person who could be central to helping a patient heal is a barrier to safe patient care. The spouse essentially threatens the nurse with a form of retaliation. Despite all these reasons that explain why the nurse in each scenario might not speak up, no excuse exists for failing to do a right thing. These scenarios exemplify what we mean when we say everyday ethical comportment.

Evidence of Failure

In 2000, the Institute of Medicine (IOM) published its groundbreaking report *To Err Is Human* (Kohn, Corrigan, & Donaldson, 1999). This report revealed that hundreds of thousands of patients might be harmed because of fundamental problems in the behavior of health care professionals. In 2005, the American Association of Critical-Care Nurses (AACN) and VitalSmarts published a landmark study, *Silence Kills* (Maxfield, Grenny, McMillan, Patterson, & Switzler, 2005). That study revealed how harmful silence can be. *Silence Kills* detailed the failures of health care professionals when it comes to having difficult conversations with colleagues. In essence, the *Silence Kills* work revealed that many of the mistakes and problems identified in the IOM report could be prevented if people would speak up when they encounter commonly occurring situations in the course of providing patient care.

The authors of *Silence Kills* describe seven situations where people fail to engage in crucial conversations (Table 3.1). These seven situations are faced consistently by health care workers, but sadly, the study found that only one in 10 health care workers will speak up when encountering them. The reasons given by participants for failing to speak up included timing (not enough or the right time), a belief that it was not their job, and fear of retaliation. The most striking finding, however, was the link between failing to speak up and four important things. Failing to speak up is associated with an increase in the number of mistakes, a decrease in the quality of patient care, a decrease in nurse-physician satisfaction, and a decrease in productivity (Maxfield et al., 2005).

Table 3.1   Situations That Health Care Providers Fail to Address

1. Broken rules

2. Lack of support

3. Mistakes

4. Incompetence

5. Poor teamwork

6. Disrespect

7. Micromanagement

Excerpted from Maxfield, Grenny, McMillan, Patterson, & Switzler, 2005.

In 2008, the Joint Commission (TJC) issued a sentinel event alert regarding behaviors that undermine patient safety (The Joint Commission, 2008a). The behaviors described in the alert represent concrete examples of disrespect in which health care workers consistently fail to speak up. In addition to bringing this critical issue to the attention of organizations via a sentinel event alert, TJC established new standards that became effective in 2009, including a code of conduct that defines acceptable and unacceptable behavior (The Joint Commission, 2008b).

In 2010, a qualitative study conducted by nurse researchers with nursing students in Florida demonstrated that the hidden curriculum reinforces the practices described in the *Silence Kills* study (Fowler Byers & Harper, 2010). In the Florida study, when nurses encountered the seven categories of crucial conversations described in the *Silence Kills* study, the nursing students observed silence. The hidden curriculum is what students learn by watching how individuals behave, rather than what they learn by being told how to behave. Nursing students observed nurses in clinical practice settings and were able to document evidence of nurses in all levels of clinical practice (direct care provider, charge nurse, and nurse manager) who failed to speak up when presented with crucial conversation opportunities. The most commonly observed situations were broken rules, disrespect, and poor teamwork, all of which are known to be linked to errors and poor quality outcomes in patient care (Kohn et al., 1999). Though the students were shocked at the circumstances, and despite being present to observe potentially harmful situations for patients, they as students did not feel it was their place to speak up. In other words, the nurses failed to intervene and thus unknowingly taught the students that remaining silent when one can prevent patients from potential harm is acceptable. This study provides some evidence that nurses learn silence even before they are independent in clinical practice (Fowler Byers & Harper, 2010).

The Association of periOperative Registered Nurses (AORN), American Association of Critical-Care Nurses (AACN), and VitalSmarts published another study, *The Silent Treatment,* that shows silence still kills (Maxfield, Grenny, Lauandero, & Groah, 2010). Nurses and other health care professionals persist in failing to take action. Nurses do not speak up when they see problems. Even with the addition of safety tools such as checklists designed to alert a team of a potential problem, 58% of respondents in this study said they were unable to speak up (Maxfield et al., 2010). The study showed that essentially "undiscussable" situations commonly occur. More than 80% of nurses in this study reported concerns about dangerous shortcuts, incompetence, and disrespect. Fewer than 35% of participants in the study reported speaking to the individual about whom they have concerns (Maxfield et al., 2010).

The data are compelling. Despite well-published studies, the creation of standards tied to certification for organizations, and multiple interventions to improve communication, poor communication, namely silence, persists as a problem for patients, health care workers, and organizations. You might ask, "How is this possible? Surely nurses, as patient advocates, would be more likely to speak up!" When silence becomes a habit in the presence of perceived wrongs, you have to wonder if our core values have eroded.

Patients and families trust that we will care for and about patients who are exquisitely vulnerable. They take it for granted that we will protect them. No nurse wants to believe that she or he would be the one to allow harm to come to a patient. Nurses must work to live the foundational core value of advocacy (American Nurses Association [ANA], 2001). When faced with an ethically challenging situation, nurses, rather than considering options in terms of "What will happen to me if I say something?" must learn to ask a different question. It isn't even as simple as, "What will happen to the patient if I fail to speak up?" Nurses must reframe their thinking and view these circumstances in terms of a moral question, "What is my moral obligation to intervene for this patient?"

Taking Action

One model of decision-making examines the impact free will has on what sort of action, if any, people take when faced with an ethics challenge (Serkerka & Bagozzi, 2007). In this model, the individual experience of emotion and considerations of competing pressures influence the action people take when faced with a moral problem. The relationship between recognizing an ethical challenge and desiring to act is mediated by the skills people believe they have and their belief in what they can do with those skills (self-efficacy). Whether or not you take action depends in part on what type of person you want to be. When faced with a moral choice, you must first possess the desire to act, then must make a decision about what type of action is consistent with who you want to be and, finally, you must take action.

When you experience an ethics challenge, you have an immediate emotional response that influences what you desire to do. People who develop an awareness of their emotional responses to ethically challenging situations can learn to regulate their response and focus more on a values motivation to formulate a plan for action. Motivations are influenced by your identity with a group (nurses, for example) and by values (personal and professional), and actions are influenced by practice. Using this model then demonstrates that moral courage, the ability to use inner values and principles to do what is good, is influenced by emotions and is a matter of practice.

 ## PURPOSE EXERCISE: CONSIDER AND WRITE YOUR ANSWERS TO THE FOLLOWING QUESTIONS

1. What are my professional goals?

2. What is my personal purpose as a nurse?

3. What impact do I want to have through my work? On whom?

4. What do I hope to accomplish as a nurse?

5. What will make my professional life worthwhile?

6. How do I want to feel about myself and my work, while I am doing it and when I am done?

The Emotional Response

Emotion plays a significant role in influencing how you act in ethically challenging situations. Emotion, more specifically caring about something, motivates you to respond in difficult situations. However, a purely emotional response, one that is not reasoned, is typically the least effective response when you are facing an ethics challenge. In the absence of reflection and self-awareness, emotions can color perceptions, which in turn can cloud judgment and impede ethical actions. A reasoned response is more likely when you develop some self-awareness and learn to reflect on circumstances rather than simply react to them. According to Serkerka and Bagozzi, emotions can enhance a cognitive process by helping an individual focus attention (2007). Imagining the desired outcome when you speak up to advocate on behalf of another can generate a positive anticipated emotional response. Instead of imagining and fearing the worst, you learn to imagine and anticipate the best. Exercising your moral imagination in this way is the practice needed to influence the desire to speak your values.

Speaking Your Values

Caring is often described as the foundation value and a central virtue for nursing. Patients surrender themselves, for the most part, to nurses who care for the patient's most intimate needs. In ethically challenging situations, nurses are expected to protect patients, even if they face some amount of personal risk. In these situations, caring is not enough to sustain or motivate nurses to do a right thing. When nurses are called to be advocates, they must integrate their personal and professional values beyond caring to define what it means to be a nurse of integrity. Nurses of integrity follow through on the spoken and unspoken promise to protect a person in a vulnerable state. Nurses must believe that advocacy is their duty: not just because it is part of the ANA code of ethics, but because it is part of who they are as people, as nurses.

It is disheartening to think that to be a nurse you have to have extraordinary courage to do what is right, because on any given day you might not feel you have it. However, courage becomes ordinary when it is practiced. Acts of courage come from habits of the heart that can be facilitated by self-reflection and regulation (Serkerka & Bagozzi, 2007). Enduring moral courage then is the ability to consistently use ethics principles and core values to do what is good for others, regardless of threats to the self.

It is hard to imagine nurses advocating on behalf of another person if they have not mastered the skill of advocating for themselves. The everyday examples discussed earlier demonstrate the subtle yet insidious nature of disrespect and how it influences the culture of the work environment nurses must navigate. When nurses fail to create, contribute to, or sustain an environment that demonstrates respect, they fail to uphold a fundamental value of ethical nursing practice (ANA, 2001). Thus, if nurses hope to advocate for patients, they must uphold their personal integrity by expecting and commanding respect from patients, their families, peers, and other members of the health care team. Like any other skill, this one needs to be practiced.

Beyond courage and the conviction that nurses have an obligation to advocate for another, nurses need communication skills at crucial moments. Few people are born with the skills necessary to speak up when they face personal risk. Just as nurses need to practice the nursing skills for starting an IV or placing a urinary catheter, they must also practice communication skills necessary to speak up in challenging situations.

Unpacking the Problem

Return to the case studies presented earlier in the chapter. Consider the following questions about each case, and write down your responses. These questions are framed to help you focus on a positive emotional response, rather than the more common potential negative one. Your ability to handle challenging situations is enhanced by your ability to make sense of the situation, to tell a positive story about it. You need to identify why something happened and to imagine what good might come from it.

Reflective Practice

1. What is the nature of the conflict in the situation?

2. What values does that conflict undermine?

3. What specific behavior communicates disrespect toward the nurse?

4. Identify a possible positive motivation for the behaviors described in the scenarios.

5. What are the benefits to the patient if the nurse chooses to address the conflict?

6. What are the potential benefits to the disrespectful person in the scenario if the nurse addresses the underlying values conflict?

6. What benefits does the nurse face if she or he openly addresses the conflict?

8. What could the nurse say that would demonstrate her commitment to underlying core values in nursing? Be specific and create a script.

Effective Speakers Learn to Listen

The standard approach to helping people learn to speak up begins with presenting steps for giving feedback. This approach is typically focused on the other person, not on the individual who is considering speaking. Perhaps a more effective strategy is to help nurses first reflect on their own behaviors by encouraging them to invite and be open to receiving feedback from others. In this way, nurses could become positive role models and leaders in changing a culture toward mutual respect.

Exercise in Receiving Feedback

The next time you are at work, reflect on how you supported the team effort for the day in caring for patients. Write down your reflections. Then ask your colleagues (nurses and other members of the team—for example, nursing assistants, physicians, housekeepers, respiratory therapists, secretaries, etc.) for feedback on how well you supported them in their efforts to provide excellent safe patient care. Don't be surprised if your invitation is met with surprise and curiosity. Be patient and persistent, and be prepared to hear how others truly perceive you. The goal of this exercise is to gain an appreciation for how others see you.

 ## PURPOSE EXERCISE: CONSIDER AND WRITE YOUR ANSWERS TO THE FOLLOWING QUESTIONS

1. Invite feedback. You may need to be specific, for example, "Did I treat you with respect? Did I follow appropriate patient care policies? Is there something I could have done better?"

2. Listen calmly and attentively. Focus on the content of what is being said, not the person delivering the message. Listen for good and bad examples of how to deliver constructive feedback to someone.

3. If you have questions, clarify the feedback.

4. Thank the other person and acknowledge their concerns. Avoid defending or overexplaining your actions.

5. Identify what was helpful to you in the way that person shared their feedback with you (e.g., positive tone; concrete, specific examples).

6. Make a commitment to meet this person at a later time and share with that person steps you have taken to address concerns. Tell her or him when you make changes that were suggested.

Exercise in Giving Feedback

After you have practiced receiving feedback, find a colleague with whom you have established a trusting relationship. Ask this colleague to participate with you in practicing giving constructive feedback. The goal of this exercise is to manage your expectations and to practice giving a colleague feedback on her or his performance. Identify a specific situation when another colleague's behavior was not consistent with what you expected. You might find it helpful to write down your thoughts before speaking with your colleague. The exercise is most fruitful if your colleague agrees to receive the feedback in the most negative way she or he can manage (for example, by yelling, being defensive, attacking you). Then work with your trusted colleague to practice what it feels like if your worst fears come true.

1. Feedback should be given only with positive intent. Focus on a common goal, for example, improving teamwork when providing patient care. In real feedback situations, the giver of feedback must mentally prepare and consider the timing of comments.

2. Describe specifically what you have observed, using facts and figures when possible. Be brief and to the point, and limit feedback to one behavior or action.

3. State the impact of the behavior or action (impact on whom). Link the behavior to goals of patient care rather than patient experience—in other words *not* patient satisfaction. Work on maintaining an objective tone in your voice.

4. Ask the other person to respond, not offer excuses. Listen objectively and, if necessary, summarize the key points.

5. Focus the discussion on solutions. If appropriate, ask specifically for the change you believe will help achieve the established goals. Leave responsibility for action with the other person (manage your expectations).

6. Ask your colleague to evaluate you on how you provided the feedback.

Other Strategies

Hopefully, after reading this chapter you will want to nurture your self-efficacy by practicing the skills necessary to make taking action possible. Practice inspires confidence in your ability to find the moral voice necessary to speak up and influence a right act in ethically challenging situations. Entire books have been written about different strategies to master becoming a skilled communicator (Patterson, Grenny,

McMillan, & Switzler, 2005a; Patterson et al., 2005b). Find one that works for you. Table 3.2 details some examples of things exceptional nurses in the *Silent Treatment* study did when confronted with "undiscussable" situations.

Table 3.2 Strategies for Success When Encountering "Undiscussable" Situations

1. When the issue is not urgent, get the facts, run pilots, work behind the scenes.

2. Assume the best and speak up; sometimes it takes just one person.

3. They explained their positive intent, helping the patient as well as the caregiver.

4. Take special effort to make it safe for the caregiver (avoid creating defensiveness).

5. Use facts and numbers as much as possible, bringing the problem individual into the situation.

6. Avoid telling negative stories or making accusations.

7. Diffuse or deflect the individual's anger.

Exemplary Practice

Nurses have remained silent in the face of ethical challenges for years. Breaking the habit of silence takes time and energy, but it does pay off. Key leaders at a New York hospital describe the process they used to establish a culture of mutual respect and, in effect, begin to break the silence (Kaplan, Mestel, & Feldman, 2010). This organization focused on two key recommendations from TJC—namely, establish a code of conduct that defines appropriate behavior, and create a process for managing behavior that undermines a culture of safety.

They created a guide to help their employees identify types of behavior that are respectful, disrespectful (uncivil or bullying), and outright bad. The guide includes examples in each of these categories and the expected response when the behavior occurs, including resources to consult. The guide was a key resource for leaders identified to pilot the initiative in the organization. Over a 3-year period, the organization showed meaningful improvements toward a culture of mutual respect. The experience of this New York organization demonstrates the step-wise approach necessary to tackle an insidious problem such as silence and takes an honest look at the challenges and successes.

Cautionary Tale: Texas Nurses

In the last few years, a very public example of when speaking up can harm nurses in their quest to do the right thing occurred in Texas. Nurses at a small Texas hospital reported their concerns about a physician to the Texas medical board. The identified physician told his friend and business partner, the local sheriff, of the report to the medical board. Over a 2-year ordeal, the nurses were eventually exonerated, but not before losing their jobs and one of them being tried on criminal charges. Eventually the physician, sheriff, hospital administrator, and prosecuting attorney all faced serious consequences for their abuse of power. The public outcry in support of the nurses was remarkable, but the events in Texas are a sad reminder that when nurses voice their values, they might face serious consequences, even when they have done the right thing to protect patients.

Undoubtedly, countless private examples of nurses experiencing retaliation when they speak up in defense of patients or personal integrity exist. It is naïve to think speaking up is a riskless endeavor. It is not, and no way to calculate the absolute risk exists. In the end, courage and support can sustain you, but that might not be enough to feed you. You are not wrong to preserve your source of income, even if you have to compromise doing the right thing. It will, however, take a toll on your integrity. Do it as a conscious choice, not an accident. Not every nurse has options to work in a different environment. Nurses as individuals can make a difference in changing an unhealthy work environment, but their power and influence are limited.

Conclusion

Ethics is, at its core, about communication. Everyday ethical behavior demands lifelong learning and regular reflection on practice. Learn to ponder the positive possibilities for giving voice to your values, particularly in ethically challenging situations. Aristotle said it best, "We are what we repeatedly do." Excellence, then, is not an act but a habit. We must practice speaking our values every chance we get. It gets easier over time.

Talk About It!

- Think about the last shift you worked. Were there any moments where you thought you should say something but did not? If you didn't say anything, what stopped you? Has it bothered you to think about it? If so, how would you do it differently if presented with the same situation again?

- Think about a specific ethically challenging situation, perhaps one from this chapter. Talk to a colleague about what you think an "ideal" nurse would do in the situation and see if your colleague describes the same behaviors.

- Is there a particular person in your work situation who makes you the most uncomfortable when you think about confronting or speaking up to him or her. Find a trusted colleague to role play, with you being yourself and your colleague the difficult person and practice how to address a complex issue with him or her. Even if you feel foolish at first, practicing this role playing will give you confidence when faced with a real situation.

References

American Nurses Association (ANA). (2001). *Code of ethics for nurses*. Washington, DC: American Nurses Association.

Benner, P., Sutphen, M., Leonard, V., & Day, L. (2010). *Educating nurses: A call for radical transformation*. San Francisco, CA: Jossey-Bass.

Fowler Byers, J., & Harper, J. G. (2010). *Student perceptions of the real world: Silence still kills*. Podium presentation, 21st Sigma Theta Tau International Nursing Research Congress, July, 2010, Orlando, FL.

Gentile, M. C. (2010). *Giving voice to values: How to speak your mind when you know what's right*. New Haven, CT: Yale University Press.

The Joint Commission. (2008a, July 9). Behaviors that undermine a culture of safety. *Sentinel Event Alert*. Retrieved from http://www.jointcommission.org/assets/1/18/SEA_40.PDF

The Joint Commission. (2008b, July 9). Leadership standard (LD.03.01.01). *Sentinel Event Alert*. Retrieved from http://www.jointcommission.org/assets/1/18/SEA_40.PDF

Kaplan, K., Mestel, P., & Feldman, D. L. (2010). Creating a culture of mutual respect. *Association of periOperative Registered Nurses*, *92*, 495-510.

Kohn, L. T., Corrigan, J. M., & Donaldson, M. S. (Eds.). (1999). *To err is human: Building a safer health system*. Washington, DC: National Academy Press.

Maxfield, D., Grenny, J., Lavandero, R., & Groah L. (2010). *The silent treatment: Why safety tools and checklists aren't enough to save lives*. VitalSmarts, AORN, & AACN. Retrieved from http://silenttreatmentstudy.com/

Maxfield, D., Grenny, J., McMillan, R., Patterson, K., & Switzler A. (2005). The seven crucial conversations for healthcare. In *Silence kills*. VitalSmarts. Retrieved from http://www.aacn.org/WD/Practice/Docs/PublicPolicy/SilenceKills.pdf

Patterson, K., Grenny, J., McMillan, R., & Switzler, A. (2005a). *Crucial confrontations: Tools for resolving broken promises, violated expectations, and bad behavior*. New York: McGraw-Hill.

Patterson, K., Grenny, J., McMillan, R., & Switzler, A. (2005b). *Crucial conversations: Tools for talking when stakes are high*. New York: McGraw-Hill.

Serkerka, L. E., & Bagozzi, R. P. (2007). Moral courage in the workplace: Moving to and from the desire and decision to act. *Business Ethics: A European Review, 16*(2), 132-149.

NURSING ETHICS IN EVERYDAY PRACTICE: USING COMMUNICATION SKILLS EFFECTIVELY

4

–Fiona Timmins, PhD, MSc, BNS RNT, FFNRCSI,
BSc Health & Soc (Open)
Associate Professor
School of Nursing and Midwifery
Trinity College Dublin

Think About It!

- Changing disease patterns and treatments; social trends; and increased population mobility, together with increasingly older population—all present ethical issues for nurses.

- Nurses need a systematic approach to dealing with ethical issues, including:

    - Identifying the situation that requires ethical consideration and decision-making

    - Reviewing relevant formal ethical standards

    - Developing alternative courses of action

    - Evaluating the alternative courses of action

    - Assuming personal responsibility for the consequences of your action

- Communication skills are essential to dealing with ethical issues effectively.

- The complexity of contemporary nursing environments, coupled with the rapid way those environments change, has made effective communication more vital for nurses than ever before.

Communication is a two-way process, involving both a sender and receiver (McCabe & Timmins, 2006). This communication can be affected and distorted by elements within either party. The way each person communicates is influenced by the environment, culture, past experiences, and understanding of the situation (McCabe & Timmins, 2006).

Nurses become experts in many forms of communication as they progress through their nursing careers. However, these communication skills are constantly being challenged and developed in response to novel situations and different sets of people. For nurses to improve their own communication skills, they need to develop self-awareness of how well they communicate with others.

This chapter is about how you as a nurse can use your communication skills effectively when you encounter ethical issues in practice. Examining your own skills in this area and increasing your self-awareness will assist you in dealing competently with any ethical issues you might face.

Challenges in Practice

Nursing practice requires a high degree of technical knowledge and a thorough understanding of your patients, their presenting disorders, and their treatments. However, nursing also requires good communication skills. Indeed, communication permeates every aspect of nursing practice and is a fundamental skill. For example, you must foster good relationships with patients and their families, explain ward routines and procedures, and provide patients with health education and advice. Communication skills are also vital in your role within the multidisciplinary team. Managing and coordinating patient care effectively without good communication are almost impossible, whether the exchange of information occurs verbally or otherwise. However, the complexity of contemporary nursing environments, coupled with the rapid way those environments change, has made effective communication more vital for nurses than ever before.

Modern nursing and health care are complex. This complexity permeates all levels of patient care but is more evident in some areas than others. Critical care units, for example, are highly technical places where patients receive specific interventions of varying complexity. Though such high levels of technology might not be evident in all areas of nursing, most cases that present in the Western world are now more complex than they were in prior decades. The whole face of the "patient" cohort is rapidly changing. Social and demographic changes, changing disease patterns and population mobility, increased complexity of care delivery and more advanced treatment solutions, and an increasingly older population all invariably present ongoing ethical issues for nurses both now and in the future.

This increasing complexity isn't the only challenge facing contemporary nurses. They also face nearly constant change. The pace of change within Western society has never been so fast. Nurses who have been in the profession for more than one generation know that tremendous changes have taken place. Health care delivery, medical interventions, medication interventions, and ways of providing nursing care changed dramatically in the past 10 years alone. Within this rapidly changing, increasingly complex environment, nurses face a range of new ethical issues associated with their practice that are also a source of stress (Ulrich et al., 2010).

Ethical issues associated with contemporary nursing and of frequent concern to contemporary nurses include the following:

- Protection of patients' rights

- Autonomy and informed consent

- Truth telling

- Indifference to a patient's presence, e.g., discussing a patient's case in front of the patient (Hughes, Hope, Reader, & Rice, 2002)

- Public embarrassment of patients

- Infantilization of patients

- End-of-life decision-making

- Initiation, withholding, and withdrawal of treatment and advance directives in acute and long-term care (Ulrich et al., 2010)

- Poor patient outcomes because of inadequate staffing

- The care of high-risk neonates

In particular, protecting patients' rights is described as one of the basic tenets of the profession (Ulrich et al., 2010). And though nurses often feel confident to address ethical issues, they also report a sense of powerlessness, a sense that they have little influence in these issues overall (Ulrich et al., 2010). What nurses need is a systematic approach to dealing with these issues and the communication skills to do this effectively.

A Systematic Approach to Ethical Decision-Making

When you are teasing out ethical issues, retaining an open mind and trying not to be influenced too much by your own personal experiences and feelings are very important. Good decision-making about what action you take, if any, to address your concerns demands sound, balanced judgment (Corey, Corey, & Haynes, 1998).

When faced with ethical issues in practice, you can use many suggested frameworks to examine your thoughts, feelings, and potential actions in the situation. Methods of dealing with ethical issues and conflicts have been covered extensively in other chapters in this book. However, broadly speaking, Pope and Vasquez (2007) suggest that some or all of the following 18 steps need to be considered when ethically complex situations arise:

1. Identify the situation that requires ethical consideration and decision-making.

2. Anticipate who will be affected by your decision.

3. Identify the client in this particular case.

4. Assess your own knowledge and competence in the area or topic. Ask yourself whether you need to improve on any relevant areas of competence, knowledge, skills, experience, or expertise.

5. Review relevant formal ethical standards.

6. Review relevant legal standards.

7. Review the relevant research and theory in the area.

8. Consider how, if at all, your personal feelings, biases, or self-interest might affect your ethical judgment and reasoning.

9. Consider what effects, if any, that social, cultural, religious, or similar factors might have on the situation and on identifying ethical responses.

10. Consider consultation with others.

11. Develop alternative courses of action.

12. Evaluate the alternative courses of action.

13. Try to adopt the perspective of each person who will be affected.

14. Decide what to do, and then review or reconsider it.

15. Act on and assume personal responsibility for your decision.

16. Evaluate the results.

17. Assume personal responsibility for the consequences of your action.

18. Consider implications for preparation, planning, and prevention.

These steps will be considered later in the chapter in the context of using and developing appropriate communication skills. A case study approach will be used to develop examples that can be used to describe the required skills. First, however, you should take a look at the fundamental principles required for good communication.

Fundamental Principles of Communication

The following are some fundamental principles of communication that will be relevant across many situations. These will be especially vital when you are communicating about sensitive ethical issues. You should:

- Be assertive and use open communication.

- Speak from your own perspective.

- Selectively disclose your feelings as appropriate.

- Always be respectful to others, regardless of how "bad" you believe the situation or deed to be.

- Avoid aggressive and manipulative communication; do not aim to put others down.

- Ensure that your body language is open and assertive. Do not raise your voice, make accusations, wag your finger, or stand over people.

- Abide by your own nursing code of conduct and the ethical principles of the organization in all communications.

- Stay within your scope of nursing practice and job description.

In all attempts to communicate, whether at a formal presentation or during a quick conversation in a hallway, awareness of your own body language is important. Even if your statements are not assertive, standing over a colleague wagging your finger would come across as aggressive. In general, in communications, an "open" posture is best. This means that you should sit or stand, where possible, at the same level as the person you are speaking with, without your arms and legs crossed (if sitting), angling your body position to mirror the other person. You need to make and retain good eye contact when you are talking, and smile to open the conversation, if appropriate.

Communicating With Patients and Family Members

You will often find it necessary to elicit information relevant to an ethical issue from patients and family members. You can help create the right environment by:

- Providing a space for discussion

- Being appropriately friendly and approachable

- Asking open questions

- Listening intently, nodding to show that you are paying attention

- Taking note of views expressed

- Not dominating the conversation

Always introduce yourself by name if you are not known to everyone who is participating in the meeting.

Arranging Meetings With Colleagues

You will also frequently be needed or requested to arrange meetings with physicians and other team members. Before and during these meetings, communication should be very respectful, aimed at relationship building. You should respect the others, especially in terms of their possible time commitments—a meeting should not be demanded, but requested, though you might need to be persistent and even adopt the "broken record" technique, discussed later in this chapter, to obtain the meeting.

Conducting a Meeting

You can begin by selectively disclosing some of your feelings related to the situation at hand, such as sadness, frustration, or disappointment. This disclosure can help set the scene and place the issue firmly as your own, rather than assigning blame and instantly placing others in a defensive stance. After the initial disclosure, you can continue by alluding to other steps you have taken regarding the situation related to ethical standards, legal advice, and social factors.

If you have communicated your views but still feel uncomfortable with the situation, reconsider the nature and type of communication. Rather than presenting at a patient case conference, consider that a confidential meeting with the physician might be best. That way neither you nor the physician will face more public exposure. In such a meeting, you might also gain further insight into the decision-making process.

Communicating Research Findings

One of the reasons you might arrange a meeting is to discuss what you have found after undertaking some research relevant to an ethically complicated issue. If this is the case, you need to communicate in a balanced way that convinces the audience of the credibility of your finds. Outlining the thorough, systematic nature of your investigations and ensuring that you use current sources (not simply your old nursing files) are important. You might need to describe how you selected and analyzed the literature and to state both the strengths and weaknesses of the findings. As you present your findings for discussion, stay open to criticism. The senior nurse or physician might have differing views or alternative literature that contradicts your views, so remain receptive to receiving new information and learning.

Remember, you cannot force your views to be accepted; all you can do is present them objectively to others.

Assertiveness and the Broken Record Technique

You might need to use assertiveness skills in some ethical situations to seek a meeting, consultation, or expert advice. For example, if you as a nurse believe it is necessary to consult with the hospital's legal adviser about a particular situation, but the senior nurse does not agree with you because she or he feels that step might escalate the situation, you should be prepared to have an assertive dialogue. The dialogue might go as follows:

> **Nurse:** "I would like to contact the hospital's legal adviser, Mrs. Z, about Mr. X's situation."
>
> **Senior nurse:** "Mrs. Z is really busy with another case, so I wouldn't disturb her right now."
>
> **Nurse:** "I know that Mrs. Z is really busy right now with the other case, but I would really like to contact her."
>
> **Senior nurse:** "Did you know that they often charge the unit a fee when we consult with her?"
>
> **Nurse:** "I know that they might charge the unit a fee, but I think that it is important to consult with her about Mr. X's case."
>
> **Senior nurse:** "They'll think that we don't know what we're doing over here if you phone them."
>
> **Nurse:** "I know that it might look as if we don't know what we're doing over here, but I really think that it is important to consult with her. I need more information in this case to help with my own decision-making."

In this assertive interaction, although the nurse received a negative response, she reiterated the same need time and time again in response to the senior nurse's reactions. In assertiveness behavior, this is known as the *broken record technique* (McCabe & Timmins, 2006). The same statement is made repeatedly until the aim is achieved or the speaker at least gets her or his point across. In the preceding example, the nurse does not become aggressive or manipulative in the response. Those behaviors would actually be less likely to succeed and could result in putting the other person down, which is not acceptable regardless of the situation. The last line, "I need more information," is also an assertive request. Using the need for more information as one of the reasons for consultation is straightforward and justified.

In a more aggressive response the nurse might say, "Well, the last time we had a situation like this, the hospital was taken to court and lost millions. Do you want that to happen?" This statement would likely elicit a totally different response from the manager and likely escalate the situation. Although from a professional perspective these responses are not appropriate for a nurse, sometimes emotions can guide our responses inappropriately. When we feel that the stakes are high, or feel some conspiracy against our views, we might think that the situation, ethical or otherwise, is so desperate that bad behavior is acceptable. However, this is not the case. From a communication perspective, nurses should always aim to be respectful of the person with whom they are communicating, whether client, family, or co-worker, while remaining assertive.

Pope and Vasquez's (2007) suggested steps, outlined above, are useful to analyze ethical issues discussed in the following case study. The discussion of these ethical issues will focus on developing communication skills that will be helpful to you in practice.

Case Study 4.1

Mrs. Jabolov, 89 years old, suffers from dementia and arthritis and is in a long-term, residential care facility. She had been living alone, supported by her daughter, until 1 year ago. At that time, following a series of chest infections, both her mobility and her general health declined. More recently at the care facility, she has suffered a series of urinary tract infections, the most recent of which does not seem to be responding to antibiotics. This morning her pyrexia rose to 39.2°C. Because she has also been experiencing increased levels of confusion and agitation and has become quite sick, the attending physician decides to transfer her to a local acute hospital to receive more intensive therapy. The nurse feels very angry about this. She feels that Mrs. Jabolov's confusion might worsen in a hospital and that she might become very upset and agitated in new surroundings. She also feels that because of Mrs. Jabolov's age and dementia, Mrs. Jabolov should be left in the long-term care facility and treated less actively. After all, if she died, her family would understand, as she no longer even recognizes them.

Reflecting on Practice

For many years now, particularly because of the work of Schön (1983), nurses have been encouraged to reflect in and on practice, to promote both personal and professional development. Using a model of reflection, such as Gibbs' model (1988), can help you develop self-awareness of your communication skills (McCabe & Timmins, 2006), understand your reactions to events, and uncover some of the associated emotions. Table 4.1 outlines the suggested phases of this model and identifies some possible responses of the nurse in the Mrs. Jabolov case.

Table 4.1   Model of Reflection in Mrs. Jabolov's Case Study

1. Describe the event.	One of my patients, Mrs. J., has dementia and is very confused. Now she is suffering from recurrent urinary tract infections, and although she has been on three antibiotics, nothing seems to be working. She has grown increasingly confused and violent over the past 24 hours and has developed a high temperature. The medical team reviewed her chart this morning and has decided to send her to a hospital for further treatment and investigations. She has not been eating and drinking, and they fear that she is becoming dehydrated.
2. Describe how it makes you feel (as a nurse).	I feel sorry for Mrs. J. and her family. She used to be a very respected school principal, and photos in her room show her when she was a glamorous woman. Right now, she looks dishevelled (no matter how hard we try to help her with her grooming). I feel very sad that she has become like this. I see that when her family members are here, she hardly recognizes them. I feel angry that the doctors are pumping medicines into her and sending her into that cold hospital to be alone and get more confused. She is old and senile anyhow—can't they just leave her alone to die here in peace? It is so frustrating.
3. Evaluate this situation. (What was good and bad about the experience?)	I'm glad Mrs. J.'s infection will be properly treated. Leaving her here with inadequate treatment would be very difficult and would cause her pain. I hate that she will be going to a hospital because this might increase her confusion.
4. Analyze the situation. (What sense can you make of it?)	I think the doctors must want to preserve life at all costs and are not really thinking of what is best for Mrs. J. At the same time, I'm glad she will get treatment. I really wish this could be done here.
5. Conclude the situation.	Overall, I feel frustrated and torn. I don't know what is best for Mrs. J. in this case.
6. Formulate an action plan. (What would you do differently in this situation, or in your future practice?)	Looking at this situation now, I think it raises serious ethical issues and that I need to consult with my supervisors about the matter and raise my concerns.

This nurse has chosen to use Gibbs' (1988) model to structure her reflection on Mrs. Jabolov's situation. This is useful to identify emergent feelings and to clarify what the emerging issues are. Without self-reflection and emotional analysis, situations like the one just described can evoke a defensive stance. In the case of Mrs. Jabolov, the nurse might be tempted to confront the doctor aggressively the next time she sees him, saying something like: "What are you doing to Mrs. Jabolov? Don't you guys know when to stop?" This, of course, would be very inappropriate and might seem unlikely. However, when emotions become entangled in the situation, reacting spontaneously and communicating in a way that puts the other person down are easy. Naturally, this can lead to defensiveness and hurt feelings on the other side (even though these might not be displayed). The doctor in question might not take kindly to being criticized, might state that you are stepping outside of your scope of practice, and might threaten to report you, suddenly escalating the situation. What can be done to prevent this?

In a situation like that of Mrs. Jabolov's nurse, you should reflect on the situation in writing before speaking with anyone. Using a reflective model table (Table 4.1) to structure these thoughts, rather than letting them run as a monologue, might be helpful. When finished with this step, you might notice, as the nurse in the preceding case did, that a myriad of feelings are involved, such as frustration, anger, and possibly sadness. Acknowledging these feelings while reflecting and perhaps when discussing the situation with colleagues can be helpful.

You need to analyze any ethical issues that arise, and examining any feelings that are stirred is best. Communication fueled by emotion might not be effective. In this case, the nurse's emotional attachment to the situation and her desire for Mrs. Jabolov to have a "comfortable death" in the long-term care unit meant that her wants and needs were opposed to those of the medical team (and possibly other staff and the family). Situations where differing wants and needs exist sometimes result in conflict. Conflict occurs naturally in nursing. Though sometimes healthy, conflict can also arise because of inadequate communication (Brinkett, 2010). The two basic types of conflict are intrapersonal conflict (conflict within oneself) and interpersonal conflict (conflict with other people; Milsted, 1996). Physician-nurse conflict centered on ethical decisions, such as those that occur during end-of-life care, is common (Brinkett, 2010).

To ensure that all communication fosters and maintains good working relationships, nurses need to make a habit of analyzing ethical issues systematically, using a framework for reflection such as the one previously discussed (Pope & Vasquez, 2007). We will now progress through this framework, using some examples from the case of Mrs. Jabolov, which was previously presented.

Framework for Reflection Steps

Step 1. Clearly Identify the Situation That Requires Ethical Consideration

The framework for reflection (Table 4.1) has already allowed us to identify the situation that requires ethical consideration and decision-making. In summary, Mrs. Jabolov requires urgent medical attention and hospitalization, but the nurse feels that this is not in Mrs. Jabolov's best interest.

Step 2. Consider Who Will Be Affected by Your Decision

The medical team might consider the fact that the nurse does not view its hospitalization decision as optimal a challenge to its collective and individual authority. Remembering that nurses' disagreements with physicians should be addressed professionally and discreetly is important, although much rhetoric exists about *medical dominance* and about nurses *unshackling themselves from medical oppression,* which has a valid theory basis (Warelow, 1996). Though aggression is a common response to conflict, nurses need to handle conflict in an assertive rather than an aggressive way, because people who feel intimidated often react defensively (Rosenblatt & Davis, 2009).

The patient and family members might also be affected by a nurse's decisions. When nurses disagree with care orders, they sometimes face a temptation to challenge the physician directly, in front of the family, patient, or both. Though nurses might be right, and indeed might bring about a change in care directive, they could undermine the physician in the patient's or family's eyes. Regardless of the differing views or arising conflict among members of the multidisciplinary team, maintaining the patient's and family's confidence in the system is of upmost importance (Wilson-Barnett, 1986). Additionally, poor staff relationships and poor communication can raise concerns among nurse managers about patient care and patient safety (Thyer, 2002).

Step 3. Figure Out Who, if Anyone, Is the Client

In Mrs. Jabolov's case, Mrs. Jabolov is clearly the client. However, the nurse also needs to consider how any actions she takes might affect Mrs. Jabolov's friends and family.

Step 4. Assess Your Relevant Areas of Competence and Identify Any Missing Knowledge, Skills, Experience, or Expertise Relating to This Situation

You might feel that as a registered nurse, you should know all the answers. However, you need to be able to admit when you do not. Being assertive, which is an important skill for nurses to learn (Timmins & McCabe, 2005), means learning that when you do not understand something, you should ask for more information. This is particularly important when ethical issues are concerned, as you are more likely to make a balanced, rational judgment if you have fully investigated the facts, rather than acting on impulse.

Step 5. Review Relevant Formal Ethical Standards

Nurses in most countries have clearly developed ethical codes to guide their practice. You should familiarize yourself directly with the content, which might be available online or from your employers. Your employers might also have ethical standards for care. In the United Kingdom (UK), the Nursing Conduct (2008) and Midwifery Council's (NMC) Code of Conduct (2008), performance and ethics provides guidance for nurses. You are also personally accountable for ensuring that you protect the interests and dignity of your patients. The code (NMC, 2008) also expects you to:

> *Work with others to protect and promote the health and well-being of those in your care, their families, and the wider community. (para. 4)*

Under this code (NMC, 2008), patients and their families ought to be involved in decision-making. Because Mrs. Jabolov might not be capable of participation, the nurse needs to ascertain the family's views about her care. A discussion with the family could take place in the presence of the multidisciplinary team and could begin with an open question such as this: "Thank you, [name/s], for taking the time to meet us today. As you know from our earlier conversations, your mother's condition is deteriorating, and we do not seem to be having any success with the various medications that have been prescribed. We are considering transferring her to the local hospital, where a consultant can investigate her condition and possibly treat her and improve it. I am wondering about your views on this. How do you feel about what we are suggesting?"

After this open question has been asked, the nurse has the family's views and can involve them in decision-making.

Step 6. Review Relevant Legal Standards

During this step, if needed, you can consult with relevant textbooks (possibly from your nurse education program), relevant clinical staff in your area, or your hospital's legal adviser.

Step 7. Review the Relevant Research and Theory

To help you further understand the situation and decide what you might do, you can examine research or theory in the area of concern. For example, Mrs. Jabolov's nurse could examine the effects of urinary infections and hospitalization in older people.

Step 8. Consider How, if at All, Your Personal Feelings, Biases, or Self-Interest Might Affect Your Ethical Judgment and Reasoning

We all can be subject to holding biases. Those biases can be based on experiences or previously held beliefs, are sometimes irrational, and are often unknown to us until we consciously reflect upon them. After you've become aware of your biases, you can avoid letting them unjustly influence your actions. (This applies to your actions in Step 7 as well, because interpretation of the literature can also easily be subject to unconscious bias.) Discussing these prejudices or feelings with a critical friend or mentor can be helpful.

Step 9. Consider What Effects, if Any, Social, Cultural, Religious, or Similar Factors Might Have on the Situation and on Identifying Ethical Responses

In this step, you expand your exploration of hidden personal biases and feelings as you account for possible social, cultural, or religious factors that could influence how you or other stakeholders view a situation. In Mrs. Jabolov's case, her family might have had religious convictions that mandated the preservation of life at all costs. A particular hospital might also have an underlying religious ethos. This does not mean that you cannot communicate your views; you can still challenge others' views in an assertive way, using the evidence you gathered in Steps 5, 6, and 7. But using this step helps you understand the social factors that influence the ethical issue's context.

Step 10. Consider Consultation

Though you might have consulted legal sources in Step 6 and the literature in Step 7, you should consider who else you might need to consult to assist your ongoing exploration of the situation. Can you speak with the physician privately about what you have discovered so far and how you feel? Sometimes being open and explaining how much the matter affects you can lead to more understanding on both sides.

From a communication perspective, you need to ensure that your consultation is with an appropriate person, adhering to your nursing code of conduct. Throughout these steps, and especially when consulting others, you must ensure that you maintain the patient's confidentiality, protect the patient's rights, and do not harm the patient (nonmaleficence). Though you might feel that exposing this situation to others will help the patient (beneficence), you need to exercise caution.

Similarly, you need to protect the rights of your co-workers and your employer. If your communication in this step exposes any of the staff publicly, for example, on a website or in a newspaper, you might inadvertently harm them. You might also harm not only this patient and her or his family, but also other patients and families, as you could substantially reduce their trust in the health care system. Your consultation in this step should be to appropriate staff, maintaining the confidentiality of the situation and the patient's rights. Any communication that could constitute "reporting" of a situation ought to be done (in later steps) using the correct local procedures, and not in an ad hoc way.

Step 11. Develop Alternative Courses of Action

After you have considered all of the previous steps, you need to decide how, why, and where you are going to communicate your views. Some suitable ways of communicating are:

- Speaking with a critical friend, mentor, or other appropriate person in confidence
- Meeting with senior staff to discuss your research in the area
- Speaking directly with the physician to discuss your feelings on the matter
- Meeting with the physician or relevant staff and presenting your case in a formal, evidence-based way.

If you feel your views are not being considered seriously, additional potential courses of action could include speaking with your manager or following policy, procedures, and guidelines to make a formal or informal complaint.

Avoid communicating your concerns directly to a patient or family, as this is likely to be outside of usual ethical standards and nursing codes of conduct. If you have strongly held views, and you believe that further action needs to be taken, always follow hospital procedures, which do not usually provide for collusion with the patient and family.

Step 12. Evaluate the Alternative Courses of Action

Before you carry out the plans you developed in Step 11, be careful to consider what the best and worst possible outcome of each action would be. In particular, consider what immediate and long-term effects your actions might have on others, and what the risks and benefits are.

In the case study, as a result of her readings, consultation, and reflections, the nurse has determined that Mrs. Jabolov's transfer to a hospital is the best course of action. However, despite now viewing the treatment as appropriate, Mrs. Jabolov's nurse still feels uneasy about it and its possible consequences, and she would like to raise these concerns.

Step 13. Try to Adopt the Perspective of Each Person Who Will Be Affected

This step elaborates on Step 12 by asking you to consider how others might feel because of your actions. This helps you to develop empathy not only for patients and their families, but also for your colleagues. All too often in these situations, countertransference of anger results in one party viewing the other party as an opponent. However, by becoming self-aware, you can begin to move away from your own biased view of the world and consider multiple perspectives.

Step 14. Decide What To Do, and Then Review or Reconsider It

At this point, you have decided on the action that you plan to take. Step 14 permits you time to reconsider whether your chosen course of action is appropriate. Although all of these steps seem to make your decision-making a lengthy process, you need to ensure that you avoid immediate, knee-jerk reactions during ethical situations.

Only when all of this thinking, reflection, and consideration have been done are you ready to go forth with your communications on the matter. Regardless of the action that you will take, some level of communication will be involved. Your options include:

- Nonverbal communication (even if you take no action)

- Verbal communication (making requests, stating views)

- Written communication (letter, report, complaint)

- Presentation

- One-to-one or team meeting

Step 15. Act on and Assume Personal Responsibility for Your Decision

In keeping with the principles of assertive communication, you must adopt a no-blame approach in these ethical situations. Dealing with the situation, moving through the steps and, possibly, taking action might be challenging. However, you have to take responsibility for your actions and the consequences. Blaming the physician, nursing staff, or hospital as you progress through the steps has a negative influence on you and prevents you from acting in an assertive way.

Avoidance is a common response to conflict, but if you believe you must take action, you must not avoid it, regardless of the consequences. Though this can be challenging for nurses, increasingly hospitals and organizations are encouraged to have supports for nurses and other staff in such situations, such as ethics committees, ethics advisers, and senior nurse mentors (Ulrich et al., 2010). However, even in the absence of such facilities, the importance of support should be recognized.

Step 16. Evaluate the Results

After you have taken action, you need to identify how successful your action was. Seek advice from relevant staff and try to establish to what extent, if at all, your action brought about the expected consequences. Identify any unforeseen consequences, as well. Decide whether, knowing what you know now, you would have acted in the same way or chosen a different response to the situation.

If your desired change in the client's situation was accomplished, this would obviously be viewed as successful. However, if it was not, do not consider your actions a failure. Perhaps you have raised awareness of the issue, or perhaps your information has provided the impetus for changing policy and practice in this regard. Examine emerging protocols and guidelines for any evidence of your actions underpinning them. You might need to be patient with this, as change generally takes time.

Step 17. Assume Personal Responsibility for the Consequences of Your Action

In the same way as Step 15, you have to take personal responsibility for consequences of any actions that you take, except now you have to evaluate the ultimate consequences of your actions rather than the immediate ones.

Step 18. Consider Implications for Preparation, Planning, and Prevention

The purpose of this chapter is primarily to consider your use of communication skills during the process of dealing with an ethical situation. To consider implications for future preparation, planning, and prevention, you might find it helpful at this point to fully examine your communications throughout the whole process using Gibbs' (1988) model of reflection (Table 4.1). Remember that your use of optimal communication skills throughout processes is vital, not only to building and sustaining relationships, but also to having a successful ethical outcome by having your voice heard.

Many government licensing organizations establish guidelines about the kind of communication skills nurses are required to have upon registration. These are the basic prerequisites for nursing practice, and you will be expected to build upon them during your career. In the UK, the Nursing and Midwifery Council (NMC) states that nurses need to demonstrate core competencies of communication and interpersonal skills (2010). The overarching requirement of competence for adult nurses is that they

…must demonstrate the ability to listen with empathy. They must be able to respond warmly and positively to people of all ages who may be anxious, distressed, or facing problems with their health and well-being (NMC, 2010, p. 15).

The NMC also describes a range of sub-competencies that nurses are expected to have:

All nurses must use the full range of communication methods, including verbal, non-verbal and written, to acquire, interpret, and record their knowledge and understanding of people's needs. They must be aware of their own values and beliefs and the impact this may have on their communication with others. (NMC, 2010, p. 15)

These examples show the regard within the profession for fundamental communication skills, such as respect and empathy. These are pivotal in all nurse communication interactions and, particularly, in keeping with this chapter's focus, when dealing with ethical issues. Thus, when you are reflecting back on the communication skills that you used during your action related to the ethical issue, consider the following:

- Did I show respect and empathy to all parties, including not just the patient and family, but also colleagues?
- Did I demonstrate warmth in my approach?
- Did my nonverbal behavior demonstrate respect?
- Did I avoid displaying aggression or hostility or raising my voice?
- Did I effectively use verbal communication skills?
- Did I fully examine my beliefs and values regarding the ethical issue?
- Was I objective and nonjudgmental with regard to the situation?
- Did I use a range of communication strategies?
- Did I behave assertively?

When you reflect and examine your communication behaviors using the preceding list, you can examine ways in which you could have been more effective and develop an action plan that you could use the next time an ethical issue arises.

Conclusion

Competence in communication is a basic prerequisite for nurses in practice. For you to develop and improve your own communication skills, self-awareness of how you communicate with others is important. This chapter considered one particular context that might challenge your communication skills: arising ethical issues in contemporary nursing practice. Communicating in these situations requires a systematic approach (Pope & Vasquez, 2007), including:

- Identifying the situation that requires ethical consideration and decision-making

- Reviewing relevant formal ethical standards

- Developing alternative courses of action

- Evaluating the alternative courses of action

- Assuming personal responsibility for the consequences of your action

Important communication skills include:

- Nonverbal communication

- Verbal communication (making requests, stating views)

- Written communication (letter, report, complaint)

- Avoiding aggressive and manipulative communication

- Using open communication

- Ensuring all your communications abide by your own nursing code of conduct and the ethical principles of the organization

- Ensuring you stay within your scope of nursing practice and job description in all communications

Remember, we are all human beings in these interactions and take with us our feelings, past experience, and education. Tipping the balance of a relationship into the negative by handling a situation badly can be very easy. That is not to say that we as nurses need to tiptoe around others, but rather that we should respond objectively and communicate with a high level of self-awareness, no matter how emotional the situation is. Communication is fundamental not just to the development of good nurse/patient relationships; it permeates almost every element of nursing practice. The absence of good communication in ethical situations can compromise patient safety and quality care delivery. As a nurse, you have a responsibility to ensure that you maintain and develop your competence in communication in the clinical environment.

Talk About It!

- How well do you communicate with others? What are the styles of communication that occur within your unit? What is your personal and professional communication style? Do they differ?

- What are the communication challenges you face in clinical practice when working through an ethical issue? What are the major barriers to good communication practices?

- Think of a clinical practice situation where your communication skills were either poorly or well-received? What were the factors that influenced this situation? If you were poorly received, what did you learn from this situation and what did you do to improve your communication skills?

- Are there specific resources that you and your colleagues readily use when faced with communication barriers with other providers, patients, and/or families?

References

Brinkett, R. (2010) A literature review of conflict communication causes, costs, benefits, and interventions in nursing. *Journal of Nursing Management, 18*(2), 145-156.

Corey, G., Corey, M. S., & Haynes, R. (1998). *Student workbook for ethics in action.* Pacific Grove, CA: Brooks/Cole.

Gibbs, G. (1988). *Learning by Doing: A guide to teaching learning methods.* Oxford, UK: Oxford Brookes University.

Hughes, J. C., Hope, T., Reader, S., & Rice, D. (2002). Dementia and ethics: The views of informal careers. *Journal of the Royal Society of Medicine, 95*(5), 242-246.

McCabe, C., & Timmins, F. (2006). *Communication skills for nursing practice.* London: Palgrave Macmillan.

Milsted, J. A. (1996). Basic tools for the orthopaedic staff nurse: Conflict management and negotiation. *Orthopaedic Nursing, 15*(2), 39-45.

Nursing and Midwifery Council. (2008). *Code of conduct.* Retrieved from http://www.nmc-uk.org/Nurses-and-midwives/The-code/The-code-in-full/

Nursing and Midwifery Council. (2010). *Standards for pre-registration nursing education.* London: Author.

Pope, K., & Vasquez, M. J. T. (2007). *Ethics in psychotherapy and counseling: A practical guide* (3rd ed.). Jossey-Bass/John Wiley.

Rosenblatt, C. L., & Davis, M. S. (2009). Effective communication techniques for managers. *Nursing Management, 40*(6), 52-54.

Schön, D. A. (1983). *The reflective practitioner: How professionals think in action.* New York: Basic Books.

Thyer, G. L. (2002). Dare to be different: Transformational leadership may hold the key to reducing the nursing shortage. *Journal of Nursing Management, 11*(2), 73-79.

Timmins, F., & McCabe, C. (2005). Nurses' and midwives' views of their assertive behaviour in workplace. *Journal of Advanced Nursing, 51*(1), 38-45.

Ulrich, C. M., Taylor, C., Soeken, K., O'Donnell, P., Farrar, A., Danis, M., & Grady, C. (2010). Everyday ethics: Ethical issues and stress in nursing. *Journal of Advanced Nursing, 66*(11), 2510-2519.

Warelow, P. J. (1996). Nurse-doctor relationships in multidisciplinary teams: Ideal or real? *International Journal of Nursing Practice, 2*(1), 33-39.

Wilson-Barnett, J. (1986). Ethical dilemmas in nursing. *Journal of Medical Ethics, 12*(3), 123-126, 135.

ETHICS CONSULTATION | 5

–Mary K. Walton, MSN, MBE, RN
Hospital of the University of Pennsylvania
Center for Bioethics, University of Pennsylvania

Think About It!

- Raising and addressing ethical concerns are professional obligations.

- Nursing colleagues are a resource; articulating ethical concerns gives them visibility and is the first step in addressing them.

- Seek to elicit the preferences and values of others. Work to understand them, rather than defending your own values.

- Ethics consultation is a valuable resource for caregivers, patients, and families in the acute care setting when ethical concerns arise in the provision of care.

Given the vulnerability of patients and the complexity of health care, nursing practice demands ethical decision-making. Nurses make decisions when providing care so frequently and so comfortably they might not recognize that these decisions reflect their personal values and the values of their profession, specialty, or practice setting. Patients trust nurses to act in their best interest at all times, especially when they are vulnerable and might be unconscious, fearful, or in pain. This trust represents a unique bond that exists between the public and the nursing profession.

Nurses advocate for patients to ensure that the care the patients receive reflects their values and preferences. Given the nature of the work of nursing, ethical concerns will inevitably arise. Nurses might feel troubled by a patient suffering seemingly without benefit, which can sometimes lead to moral uncertainty and moral distress. Patients and their surrogates have the authority to consent to or refuse treatments. However, physicians control many aspects of care by virtue of their place in the medical hierarchy, and by legal and regulatory requirements for medication orders and other interventions. As a result, nurses often feel compromised with respect to decision-making by and for patients who are critically ill and unlikely to survive. In these situations, they are often "in the middle" between the patient and the physician or other organizational aspects of care (Hamric, 2001; Murphy, 1993).

Nurses describe enacting their moral agency "within a shifting moral context; working in-between their own identities and values and those of the organizations in which they worked; working in-between their own values and the values of others; and working in-between competing values and interests" (Varcoe et al., 2004, p. 319). Nurses thus situated might be hesitant to bring ethical concerns forward, given the power dynamics and competing loyalties in the workplace. Moral dilemmas can arise from the complexity of the care options available and the need to reconcile those options with prevailing cultural values. Uncertainty about the right course of action prompts this question: What is the right thing to do, and what makes it so? A situation where the right action is recognized but cannot be enacted also creates moral distress. The cases studies below illustrate ethical concerns that might present to practicing nurses, trouble them, and prompt them to seek help from organizational resources, such as the ethics consultation service. Clinical ethics consultation is an established, available, and accessible resource to bedside nurses in most practice settings.

Case Study 5.1

The nurse manager of the cardiothoracic surgical intensive care unit (CTSICU) pages the ethics consultation beeper. The nurse caring for the patient today requests a consultation about a long-term patient who is under her direct care for the first time. During the past week, several staff nurses requested not to be assigned to the care of this patient, who has been in the unit for several months. Can ethics help?

The patient, Mr. Thornton, is 59 years old with history of coronary artery disease, stage IV ischemic cardiomyopathy, and diabetes. A ventricular assist device (VAD) was placed 8 months ago, and the patient received a heart transplant 4 months ago. Mr. Thornton has been hospitalized in the CTSICU since the transplant. The patient had a tracheostomy and gastrostomy placed for ventilatory and nutritional support months ago, and his course has been complicated by GI bleeds, recurrent sepsis with resistant organisms, peritonitis, and now emerging renal and hepatic dysfunction. Acute renal failure required the initiation of dialysis 4 weeks ago. His wife initially visited daily, but for the past month has been visiting only every 3 or 4 days. The patient is intermittently responsive to painful interventions and at times can nod, seeming to indicate a response to questions. Critical care attending physicians rotate every 7 days, and CT surgeons, transplant service, infectious disease, renal, and clinical nutrition consult or follow Mr. Thornton's care. Direct communication with the patient is difficult and at times not possible. The patient's wife refused to authorize a Do Not Resuscitate (DNR) order when the issue was broached by critical care attending physicians, stating that her husband wanted a transplant and indicated that he wanted all interventions possible in order to survive. The nurses describe their care as "torturing" him, offering as evidence the patient's "silent scream" when touched. They ask that ethics weigh in on what the goals of care should be, given their assessment that further interventions are medically futile, and the nursing care induces pain and suffering with no hope for recovery and an inevitable death.

Case Study 5.2

The night shift nurse text-pages the ethics beeper at 3 a.m.: *"Please call the RN caring for Mrs. Armondt during the day,"* after providing extensive wound care for a 50-year-old woman in postesophagectomy status for cancer. Her postoperative course has been rocky and required placement of a tracheostomy for long-term ventilatory support. The patient has a J-tube for nutrition, as well as signs of emerging liver and renal failure. Her surgeon is optimistic given the surgical outcome and her survival of past bouts of sepsis. Her spouse and children desperately want her to live. They have been able to visit only infrequently over this second and third month of hospitalization because of family responsibilities and the 3-hour drive to the academic medical center. Renal failure is deemed permanent, and dialysis will be an ongoing necessity. However, the surgeon offers daily encouragement during rounds. The RN relates to the ethicist that the patient repeatedly mouths to the nurse, "I want this to stop," "I want to die," and "I have had enough." Although the nurses document the patient's statements and share them verbally with physicians and family members, the physicians do not respond when nurses present the statements in rounds. Critical care physicians defer to the primary surgical team for long-term management issues. Family members' responses to nurses relating the patient's statements are either silence or replies of, "She cannot give up now." The nurses who have heard the patient's pleas to stop want to know, "Can ethics help?"

Case Study 5.3

An elderly woman has been a patient in the medical intensive care unit for 6 months with heart failure. When alert, Ms. Woodland is quiet and accepting of nursing care. Her children's visits are increasingly infrequent. Phone calls to the unit are no longer daily, and voice messages left by staff to notify family of changes in condition are not returned. Now the patient requires support for pulmonary and renal function. Ms. Woodland does not have an advance directive. Early in the hospitalization, she deferred to her sons for all medical decisions. Physicians approached the sons a month ago and recommended a DNR order in the event of cardiac arrest, but the sons adamantly demanded that all aggressive care be given to their mother. The nurses spend hours in her room each shift managing multiple infusions and technical devices to support the failing organ systems, and interventions to protect her fragile skin stressed by the pressure of interstitial fluid and immobility are intensive. Although she is somewhat responsive at times and "stable" with continuing aggressive support, neither her physicians nor her nurses expect her to improve, let alone survive to be discharged from intensive care. The patient's body is swollen and her skin tense with interstitial fluid. Managing just her skin care is overwhelming at times. Nurses and physicians remark on the patient's visible bodily deterioration and wonder what would be the most ethical way to proceed.

What Is Ethics Consultation?

Ethics consultation (EC), also known as health care or clinical ethics consultation, is defined as:

> *A set of services provided by an individual or group in response to questions from patients, families, surrogates, health care professionals, or other involved parties who seek to resolve uncertainty or conflict regarding value-laden concerns that emerge in health care (ASBH, 2011). Moral concerns presented for EC will vary and the relevant goals may include*
>
> - *To help clarify and articulate the patients' preferences,*
> - *To bridge the gap between patients' preferences and reality when there is a discrepancy,*
> - *To ensure respect for individuals' values among not only patients and their families, but providers as well,*
> - *To reduce moral distress among all parties, [and]*
> - *To optimize good decision-making*
>
> *(Craig & May, 2006, p. 170)*

Ethics consultation is typically one of the three functions of hospital-based ethics committees, along with staff education and policy development (Aulisio & Arnold, 2008). A recent national survey of U.S. general hospitals revealed that 81% had ethics consultation services and an additional 14% were in the process of developing them (Fox, Myers, & Pearlman, 2007). The need for such a consultation service is evident, considering the complexity of health care decision-making and the diversity of individual values. Furthermore, there is a growing recognition of the rights of individuals and the implications of those rights for health care. The need for this service is recognized in national standards for quality. Hospitals accredited by The Joint Commission are required to have and use a "process that allows staff, patients, and families to address ethical issues or issues prone to conflict" (The Joint Commission, 2011, LD.04.02.03; EP 2, 3). Organizations seeking designation as a Magnet organization by the American Nurses Credentialing Center (ANCC) must describe and demonstrate how nurses use available resources to address complex ethical issues (ANCC, 2008). Within critical care, the American Association of Critical-Care Nurses (AACN) Beacon Award for Excellence requires a description of how critical care units identify and resolve care-related ethical issues and how unit leaders identify and manage issues that create moral distress (AACN, 2011).

Variation in ethics consultation is well-recognized (Fox, Myers, & Pearlman, 2007). Consultants' backgrounds, preparations, and experiences are typically diverse. Assessing quality is challenging in most programs across practice settings. As a result, over the past few years a movement has developed for standardization and a process for certification or credentialing of ethics consultants. The American Society for Bioethics and Humanities publishes core competencies and is leading this movement. Given the variability in practice, the Clinical Ethics Credentialing Project incorporated elements from literature and practice to describe the fundamental elements of a clinical ethics consultation (CEC) as an intervention in which a trained clinical ethics professional:

- *Responds in a timely fashion to the request for a CEC from any member of the medical care team, patient, or family member;*

- *Reviews the patient's medical record;*

- *Either interviews relevant medical stakeholders or gathers the clinical care team and other consultants to discuss the case;*

- *Visits the patient and family whenever possible;*

- *As a preliminary matter, identifies the ethical issues at play and any sources of conflict;*

- *Involves the patient or family with care providers to promote communication, explore options, and seek consensus, when appropriate;*

- *Employs expert discussion of bioethical principles, practices, and norms and uses reason, facilitation, negotiation, or mediation to seek a common judgment regarding a plan of care going forward;*

- *Attends to the social, psychological, and spiritual issues that are often at play in disagreements about the proper course of care;*

- *Triggers a further process with hospital medical leaders or a bioethics committee to resolve the situation, if a resolution is not reached;*

- *Follows up with a patient and family after the initial consultation (although this feature of CEC varies, since in some systems follow-up is a task solely for the medical team);*

- *Records the process and substance of the consultation, including the consultant's recommendations and their justification, as part of the patient's medical record;*

- *Reviews the consultation with others on the CEC service as a basic level of evaluation and peer review; and*

- *Utilizes a formal and rigorous quality improvement process.*

(Dubler et al., 2009, p. 25).

Various approaches to EC over the last 30 years are described in the bioethics literature and range from an individual ethicist taking an authoritative role in a case to a group of individuals facilitating consensus based on ethical principles (ASBH, 2011). Nurses are among the individuals who perform ethics consultations, along with physicians, social workers, chaplains, administrators, and attorneys. The majority (91%) of general hospitals represented in the national survey reported nurses serving in this role (Fox et al., 2007).

Familiarity with the organizational approach to ethical concerns, the composition of the ethics committee, and the consultation process promotes staff knowledge of and comfort with ethics consultation. Although an orientation to organizational resources and processes to address ethical issues is mandated by The Joint Commission, the visibility of the service varies with practice settings and the activity of the service (The Joint Commission, 2011, CAMH, HR.01.04.01 EP 6). Educational venues such as grand rounds, inservice programs, and journal clubs offer a safe way to illustrate the approach used and might help avoid a negative perception of moral scrutiny. Requests for presentations to practice groups by ethics committee members and, in particular, nurse members of the consult service are usually welcomed. Discuss the kinds of ethical concerns that colleagues bring forward to the service and how the concerns are addressed. Developing a relationship with the ethics consultants can give visibility to ethical concerns without necessarily requesting a formal consultation. Using cases from the literature can foster discussion about the values at play and how to address the moral concerns and conflicts illustrated in the narrative. Developing knowledge of resources and familiarity with consultants might empower staff to recognize moral concerns and seek to address and resolve them.

Access to Ethics Consultation

All health care providers as well as patients, families, and surrogates should have access to EC services (ASBH, 2011). Almost all EC services (95%) report that anyone can request a consultation (Fox et al., 2007). First, know your organization's policies and procedures on ethics consultation, including the process for initiation and any prerequisites for the requester. Some organizations require either permission from or consultation with the patient's attending physician prior to initiating a consultation. Others mandate that the official request be submitted by a manager rather than a frontline staff person. These requirements might represent a supportive or, alternatively, a restrictive process. Sharing an ethical concern with a clinician or manager familiar with the situation might provide another perspective, relevant information, additional resources, or validation of the concern. Frontline staff distressed by a care situation often benefit from sharing the concern. Giving voice to the moral concern by organizing the information, presenting it, and answering the listener's questions is a valuable first step in addressing the issue. Frontline staff should never be restricted from taking an individual ethical concern forward for ethics consultation, whether or not others share the concern or identify the issue as value-laden. Nurse managers should always support bedside nurses in consulting the ethics service.

Although nurses might have direct access to the EC service based on policy, they might face deterrents to the decision to request a consultation. One study of nurses' experience with ethics consultation found that nurses lacked knowledge of the service or were hindered from accessing this resource by the power dynamics of the practice setting (Gordon & Hamric, 2006). The investigators suggest that it should not require an act of courage for a health care professional to raise an ethical concern or question. Nurses should know the policy and procedures for initiating a consult and follow them. These documents are developed to inform and help staff initiate what could be an unfamiliar process. Nurses could query colleagues to discover any relevant patterns or history of ethics consultations. Have they been helpful? If not, ask why.

But also note that the frequency of consultation and staff familiarity with EC might not necessarily indicate the quality of the service or staff satisfaction with it. For example, in practice settings where ethical questions and concerns are openly discussed and addressed along with other aspects of clinical care, the need for ethics consultation might be infrequent. On the other hand, few consults could represent the suppression of ethical concerns, with a request being made only when the situation becomes highly charged with open conflict among caregivers, patients, families, and surrogates. Staff satisfaction might be influenced by whether the outcome is consistent with staff preferences and values rather than those of the patient.

The Advocacy Role of the Nurse

Given the nature of their work, nurses are well positioned to recognize value-laden concerns that arise in health care. These concerns might be those of the nurse, patient, family, or any member of the clinical care team. Values, strongly held beliefs, ideals, principles, and standards inform nursing practice and ethical decision-making. Values might be individually held, or they might be grounded in professional codes or culture. "The relationship between nurse and the patient occurs within the context of the values and beliefs of the patient and the nurse" (American Nurses Association, 2010, p. 6). After extensive review of the nursing literature on patient advocacy, nurse researchers offer the view of patient advocacy as "a process or a strategy consisting of a series of specific actions for preserving, representing and/or safeguarding patients' rights, best interests, and values in the healthcare system" (Bu & Jezewski, 2006, p. 107). Ethics consultation is one process that nurses can initiate to advocate for a patient. Nurses might also initiate a consult relating to preserving their own integrity.

In addition to requiring expert knowledge and technical skill, nursing practice is governed by the values embedded in the American Nurses Association *Code of Ethics*. Revisions to the code reflect the changing roles of nurses and their relationships with colleagues. The code informs nurses, other health professionals, and the public of nursing's central values (ANA, 2008). It also is a useful framework for considering ethical concerns, identifying professional obligations, and determining the right course of action. The central ethical values, duties, and commitments embedded in the ANA *Code of Ethics* (2008) can guide nurses in determining if a concern is an ethical one and identifying professional obligations that necessitate action.

Preparing to Initiate a Consultation

What are value-laden concerns in health care that trouble nurses and prompt ethics consultations? Consider ANA's definition of nursing: "Nursing is the protection, promotion, and optimization of health and abilities, prevention of illness and injury, alleviation of suffering through the diagnosis and treatment of human response, and advocacy in the care of individuals, families, communities, and populations" (ANA, 2010). The values of the profession are evident in this definition. Core values of the profession are also embedded in the American Nurses Association *Code of Ethics*. Consider provisions articulating that the "primary commitment is to the patient, whether an individual, family, group, or community," but that you have duties to yourself as well, including "the responsibility to preserve integrity" (ANA, 2001). The Ethics Resource Center (2009), a nonprofit research organization, offers a list of values (http://www.ethics.org/resource/definitions-values) on its website that might underlie a concern or conflict. The list, which defines values ranging from acceptance to wisdom, can be a useful tool to promote reflection and discussion.

- **Commitment:** Being bound emotionally or intellectually to a course of action or to another person or persons.

- **Community:** Sharing, participation, and fellowship with others.

- **Compassion:** Deep awareness of the suffering of others coupled with the wish to relieve it.
- **Flexibility:** Responsive to change.
- **Gratitude:** A feeling of thankfulness and appreciation.
- **Hardworking:** Industrious and tireless.
- **Honesty:** Fairness and straightforwardness of conduct.
- **Honor:** Principled uprightness of character; personal integrity.
- **Hope:** The feeling that something desired can be had or will happen.
- **Humility:** Feeling that you have no special importance that makes you better than others.
- **Optimism:** A bright, hopeful view and expectation of the best possible outcome.
- **Patience:** The ability to accept delay, suffering, or annoyance without complaint or anger.
- **Reconciliation:** Enabling two people or groups to adjust the way they think about divergent ideas or positions so they can accept both.
- **Reliability:** Consistent performance upon which you can depend or trust.

Pain Management

The challenge of treating pain, particularly in end-of-life care, can create conflict because of different philosophies surrounding pain management and how best to alleviate perceived suffering. For example, physicians might resist ordering opioids based on organ function or preservation. Likewise, pharmacists might object to dispensing what they consider to be extreme doses of opioids. The nurse at the bedside might simply want relief for her patient's pain and ask, "Why is the patient suffering like this?" At times, patients might request relief to the nurse and then defer to family members who oppose medicating for pain because of their fear of hastening death or their desire for the patient to remain alert and communicative. Patients and family members might even view suffering as redemptive. Additionally, on a practical level, protocols governing the use of venous access lines to prevent bloodstream infections might inhibit treatment of pain. Clinicians must balance access for pain medication among competing infusions of chemotherapy, antibiotics, and nutrition.

In any one patient care scenario, the competing values of stakeholders might create uncomfortable and distressing situations for the nurses, yet all parties involved care about the patient and can be viewed as having the patient's best interest as paramount.

Confidentiality

Personal as well as professional values come into play in health care, producing conflict. Consider the critical care nurse who promises a patient that his or her status for human immunodeficiency virus and illegal drug use will not be revealed to family. When the patient subsequently becomes unresponsive and a family member as the surrogate decision-maker seeks information, the values of honesty, confidentiality, and informed consent create conflict for the nurse. The nurse must consider the promise to the patient to not reveal information, as well as the considerations for informed consent. Does the surrogate decision maker need to know the information in order to make decisions? If the patient recovers, the fact that the nurse honors the promise of confidentiality will likely impact the patient's trust in health care providers.

Respect for Autonomy

An individual's cultural values also influence health care. Western biomedicine places a high value on the individual's right to make autonomous decisions. Many other cultures value family, community, or elder decision-making processes. Conflict might result when clinicians resist communicating with people other than the patient or fail to allow time for this communication to occur. These cultural variations in how health care decisions are made can produce value-laden conflict.

Whose Concerns Are Being Presented?

Ethics consultation can address the concerns and values of the patient, nurse, family, or clinical team. When preparing to initiate a consult:

- Be clear on whose concern is being brought forward.

- Whose values are at play in the situation? Who shares them?

- What are conflicting values that others might hold? What is their role in the situation?

- Are the patient and family values evident?

- Was the hospitalization sudden or due to chronic condition?

- Are specialty values in conflict with those of the patient or family?

Nurse ethicist Ann Baile Hamric believes that as a moral concept, "Advocacy requires the nurse to actively support patients in speaking up for their rights and choices, in helping patients to clarify their decisions, in furthering their legitimate interests, and protecting their basic rights as persons, such as privacy and autonomy in decision making" (Hamric, 2000, p. 103).

Nurses appreciate that family members might have heard a variety of perspectives from the different providers they've dealt with during their loved one's care. The perspective of a physician working in an intensive care unit might differ significantly from that of the oncologist or the surgeon. What do family members already know? What do they need to know? Have they had other experiences with intensive care, cancer, trauma, and life-threatening illnesses? What experiences have informed their understanding and satisfaction with how decisions are being made? Was this hospitalization sudden or one of many because of an underlying chronic condition?

The nurse is often the first professional to recognize that the patient or family has a value-laden concern. Conversations at the bedside over the course of the hospitalization might reveal patient and family values, culture, and experience of care. Nurses work with the patient and family to assess their understanding of the diagnosis, treatment plan, rationale, risks, and benefits. These conversations provide the opportunity to recognize confusion, discomfort, or dissatisfaction with the plan of care, communication, or decision-making. Patients and family members might share misgivings about or dissatisfactions with the treatment plan, either in the presence of the nurse or directly with the nurse, but their values might not be evident to the physicians. Thus, the nurse might recognize and be troubled by a value conflict that is invisible to other members of the team. Nurses must determine how best to advocate for the patient among the options of care conferences, family meetings, and the like or when to request assistance from the ethics consultation service or team.

Be sure to consider patients and family members who value information and detailed discussion about all care options and want time to process information through sharing with a network of family and friends. Those patients and family members might find their active participation in learning about and understanding treatment options hindered by health literacy, language barriers, and competing home or work responsibilities, among other variables. Although informed consent is a well-established value in U.S. hospitals, patients and families often face structures and processes for care that do not always facilitate it. Consent documents are often long and filled with dense legal terms they do not understand. And their efforts to establish a trusting relationship with care providers might be hindered by lack of continuity of medical and nursing care. Family meetings to foster shared decision-making are not often held unless conflict is expected, or the family or patient resists medical recommendations. Nurses are in a unique position to help patients and families navigate past these barriers.

Nurses might have ethical concerns of their own relating to either professional or personal values, and they might face moral decisions in their daily practice. As advances in science and technology introduce new interventions, nurses grapple with the moral implications of participating in emerging practices. Organ procurement after the circulatory determination of death, deactivation or explantation of cardiovascular devices, and selective termination or reduction in multiple pregnancies are all recognized as ethical and legally permissible, yet these situations require each nurse, as a moral agent, to reflect on personal values and beliefs to determine whether her or his participation is morally acceptable. An ethics consultation might be an effective forum to address the moral considerations of the nursing staff while honoring obligations to care for the patient and family. Personal values relating to spiritual or other moral considerations might prompt a nurse to request not to care for a specific patient or participate in a certain care practice as a conscientious objection. In some organizations, the ethics committee or consultant reviews requests to opt out of specific aspects of clinical care for ethical or spiritual reasons.

An Example: The Patient Who Refuses a Recommendation for Surgery

A patient who has repeatedly refused the medical recommendation for limb amputation after careful discussion of the risks and benefits shares with the bedside nurse that she feels not just pressured, but *coerced* into giving consent. The nurse is troubled, despite the belief that the amputation is in the patient's best interest from a purely physiological perspective. The interpretive statements related to Provision One of the ANA *Code of Ethics* reveal the patient's right to self-determination and the nurse's obligation to preserve and protect that right (ANA, 2001). Although the nurse supports the medical recommendation, the nurse's obligation is to respect the patient's values and the principle of informed consent, although she might face negative reactions from colleagues who value efficiency in addition to informed consent. The nurse might identify the ethics consultation service as a resource to assist both the patient and the clinical team with the decision-making. This process might reveal deeper understandings of the patient's explanatory framework. The clinical team might discover approaches to overturn the patient's refusal or, alternately, understand and respect the patient's values and preference. Ultimately, the patient has the authority to reject recommendations, and the team is obligated to respect the patient's wishes.

When the patient, family, and clinical team are all in agreement with the decision-making process and plan of care, they have no need for an ethical consultation.

Presenting Your Concern

Although ethics consultation services have been a recognized resource in most acute care practice settings for several decades, nurses' reluctance to bring a concern forward and fear of retaliation are reported in the literature (Danis et al., 2008; DeWolf Bosek, 2009; Gordon & Hamric, 2006). This reluctance is understandable, given the hierarchical culture of medicine and the sensitivity about values in health care. If one member of the care team is uncertain about the rightness of a treatment plan or perceives that a patient's rights are being violated, the implication is that another member of the team is doing something wrong or is participating in the violation of rights. Furthermore, the moral concerns that arise in nursing practice might not be meaningful for other members of the health care team. The family or clinical team might remain committed to continue aggressive care while the bedside critical care nurse recognizes its physiological futility, causing moral concerns. These moral concerns might relate to the deterioration of the body, the infliction of pain without benefit, and the nurse's perceived position of powerlessness.

Patients dependent on technology require the intensive surveillance and interventions provided by the nurse, who might spend the entire 8 to 12 hours of a shift at the bedside of one patient. Additionally, the nurse might establish a relationship with the family and develop a deep understanding of their values, preferences, and suffering. As the physicians and other team members do not have this much exposure to the patient or family, they might not observe or appreciate the extent of the patient's pain and suffering or the value-laden concerns arising from the care. These worries might deepen nurses' moral concerns about participating in care felt to be nonbeneficial.

Gathering more information from family and colleagues helps to clarify the values at play and other stakeholders' understanding of the issue. After a value-laden concern or conflict is recognized, an important first step is to give voice to the concern, seek more information, and possibly identify others who share or can validate your concern. Present the concern to a colleague, framing the problem and positioning it as an opportunity for learning rather than a reproach. Start with questions rather than assertions. Recognize any shared values and goals (Gentile, 2010). Compare these two expressions of concern about a plan to return a critically ill patient to surgery:

- "I cannot believe the plan is to take this patient back to the operating room! This is futile."

- "I am as worried about this patient's prognosis as I imagine you are. Can you tell me more about the decision for surgery? I am interested in understanding more about the plan of care."

When nurses suppress concerns until feelings of frustration and anger develop, the recipient of the concern might hear the message as an expression of anger. This might prompt defensiveness rather than a sharing of information or a validation of the nurse's concern. Understanding the medical perspective and goals of care is an important aspect of initiating an ethics consultation related to a particular patient's care.

Initiating a Consultation

Presenting an ethical concern about the values reflected in a patient's care to an individual outside of the care team requires thoughtful preparation. How the concern is presented influences how the ethics consultant perceives the question or problem:

- Identify the pertinent information and reflect on how to present the information. In essence, think about how to tell the story and where to start. Are you presenting a personal ethical concern or bringing the concern of another to the ethics consultant?

- Be prepared to provide preliminary information to the ethics consultant. Many services have a standard intake process to aid the consultant in identifying the ethical concern and key stakeholders and begin to plan how to respond to the request. Basic intake information typically includes the following:

  - The requestor's contact information and role

  - The urgency of the request

  - Brief description of the case and the ethical concerns as the requestor understands them

  - Any steps taken to resolve the concerns

  - The type of assistance required—for example, a forum for discussion, policy interpretation, or conflict resolution

  - The key stakeholders

  - The attending physician's awareness of the ethics consult

Consider the following two versions of an initial consultation request. The scenarios are intended to offer examples of how a nurse might talk with an ethics service consultant in an initial request or intake.

> "I am a staff nurse in the surgical intensive care unit. One of our patients is being tortured with overly aggressive care. She is going to die. All the nurses feel the way I do—or they should—but I am the only one who will take the risk of calling ethics. As far as I can tell, her family and her surgical team have abandoned her. Ethics should do something to stop this. I do whatever I can to avoid being assigned to her care, as I cannot stand to cause this woman to suffer. I should not have to put up with this. Can you do something about this situation?"

> "I am a staff nurse in the surgical intensive care unit caring for Ms. A. B. I have been caring for her consistently over the past several months. My assessment is that this patient will never recover sufficiently to leave the intensive care unit. Her suffering seems without any hope of benefit, and we have done all we can to maximize her pain management. The family is unable to visit much. I am concerned that they do not have an accurate understanding of either her intense suffering or her prognosis. The surgical care team continues to be hopeful, although I do not think they appreciate her level of suffering and physical pain, either. I am troubled by participating in her care and causing such suffering that appears to me without benefit. A number of my nursing colleagues share

my feelings. I have reviewed the staff rights policy and know that I could invoke my right not to participate in her care any longer, yet that feels like abandoning my patient. I know this patient well and believe I have a professional obligation to bring my concern forward. Could you help us look at the ethical issues—perhaps in a care conference? I think we need to review the goals of care and evaluate progress to date. I approached the attending surgeon, but she does not share my concerns, and she strongly believes there is a chance of recovery with the current treatment approach, with discharge to an extended care facility. I let her know that I planned to request an ethics consultation. I think she understands my distress."

These presentations both convey the concern of the nurse. However, the second more clearly conveys recognition of the professional obligations as well as some preliminary information gathering. What are the nursing values that are embedded in this clinical situation? What are the obligations of the nurse to the patient, family, and care team, and to self? How clearly are they articulated? How might an ethics consultant vary in responding based on the difference in the initial presentations?

The ethics consultant must determine if the request represents an ethical concern. The requestor should answer all the intake questions as well as possible. Recognize that questions reflect the consultant's desire to understand the context and begin to gather facts. Some questions might not be immediately answerable. Some requests for assistance should be handled by other offices or resources—for example, legal questions, allegations of misconduct or impaired practice, or patient care complaints. Consider the consultant's questions for more information and details as an essential part of the process to understand the concern, clarify the request, and provide the appropriate response. It is not meant to be intimidating or challenging. The question-and-answer conversation often helps to reveal important considerations.

Formulating an Ethics Question

One standardized approach to ethics consultation developed in the Veterans Health Administration (VHA) and subsequently adopted by other organizations includes formulating an ethics question in one of these two structures:

- Given (*uncertainty or conflict about values*), what decisions or actions are ethically justifiable?

- Given (*uncertainly or conflict about values*), is it ethically justifiable to (*decisions or action*)?

Formulating an ethics question with the initial request helps both the consultant and the requestor to focus on the values at play and to plan the subsequent steps (Fox, Berkowitz, Chanko, & Powell, 2006). The consultant might query how the consent for surgery was obtained, the family members' understanding of the goals of care, and details about the conversation between the nurse and the physician. Examples of initial formulation of the ethics question for this example include:

- Given the conflict between the family's legal right to give consent for surgery on behalf of the patient and the nurse's obligation to act in the best interest of the patient, what decisions or actions are ethically justifiable?

- Given the family's right to give consent for surgery and the nurse's belief that the patient is dying and palliative care is indicated, is it ethically justifiable for the nurse to refuse to care for the patient? Is it ethically justifiable to perform surgery on the patient? Is it ethically justifiable to continue with aggressive intensive care, including surgery?

The details and context shape the formulation of questions. Questions formed might be numerous, and often the consultant and requestor can identify several ethically justifiable options. As the consultation evolves, the formulation of the ethics question might change. The ethics consultant works with the requestor to determine the urgency. Ethics consultations need to gather information from the patient, family, clinicians, and medical record.

Ethics consultants often characterize their work as "slowing the decision-making process down" for all parties to be heard and to listen. Thus, unless the request for assistance can be satisfied with an answer to a question or a straightforward policy interpretation, the consultation evolves over a day, a week, or even longer, depending upon the nature of the concern and the complexity of the situation. Ethics consultants are knowledgeable about basic legal aspects of health care decision-making and organizational human resource policies. Many ethical concerns have legal issues entwined. Consultants can gather information and consult with the organization's general counsel to address legal questions regarding consent, guardianship, advance directives, and other legal aspects as they arise in the consultation. For some consultations, a separate legal analysis of the questions is necessary. Recognize that ethical and legal analyses of clinical problems are distinct and may render different responses or recommendations. Consult the hospital's general counsel for expert advice on the legal considerations or ramifications of the issue.

Nurses believing that providing a dying patient with continued aggressive intervention that is causing pain and suffering is unethical might be working with a medical team, patient, and family who believe that continued care is the right thing to do. In this situation, reflecting on personal values and reviewing organizational policies on staff rights might help nurses in articulating their concern. Conscientious objection to participating in certain clinical care activities based on moral considerations is a professional obligation.

The Nurse's Role and Responsibilities—Consultation

After the ethics consultant accepts the request for the consultation based on an ethical concern or conflict, nurses are key allies for assisting in the process.

Identify the Key Stakeholders

The nurse might recognize stakeholders that the consultant should involve in the process. For example, the nurse requesting the consult might know that a resident physician on a previous rotation established an effective working relationship with the patient and family during a care crisis. A night shift nurse, a respiratory therapist, or the patient's neighbor might bring an important perspective to the consultant as well.

Illustrate the Patient's Daily Life

Concerns about the patient's quality of life might arise in ethical discussions. Only the patient can evaluate the quality of his or her life. However, a description of the patient's experience of care in a hospital setting is invaluable for most ethics consultations. Nurses with 24-hour-a-day bedside responsibilities for surveillance and care can give witness to the patient's experience.

Understanding the patient's story beyond that of the immediate issue or decision helps to support a decision-making process that respects the patient's preferences and values. Important questions might include the following: Does the patient experience pleasure? Does music or a television provide pleasant diversion from pain or boredom? How does the patient respond to care? Treatments that appear minimally invasive to clinicians can prompt distress and suffering. If interventions such as subcutaneous injections, enteral feedings, turning, and suctioning provoke negative reactions, that suffering might be relevant, yet not visible to the consultant. What is the level and intensity of the patient's pain? Has the patient expressed feelings in the middle of the night to a bedside caregiver? Does the patient seem to find daily life satisfying? Who cares for the patient? How does the patient relate to family at the bedside? Does anyone call to ask about the patient? These details provide context and give shape to the patient's perspective and interests.

Support the Patient and Family

As unfamiliar as ethics consultation might be to nurses, it might be even more so to the patient and his or her family. This is most likely a once in a lifetime experience at a critical time in a family's life. Illness or trauma causing hospitalization is a major life disruption. The fear of the unknown or the evolving disease trajectory where disability or even death hovers might be incapacitating to the patient and the family and inhibit communication and decision-making. Patients and families are burdened as they struggle with determining the right thing to do. These decisions might have significant consequences in terms of suffering, loss, and grief. Financial considerations and other outcomes of decisions might also weigh heavily on families. This is a time for empathy, kindness, and support. A nurse who has established a relationship with the patient and family may be able to offer this during this intense time.

As needed, facilitate the consultant meeting with the patient and family. Introduction by the nurse might provide comfort to the patient and the family. Some consultants do not have a clinical background, whereas others who are clinicians by training might be comfortable in an intensive care situation. If assistance with communication is needed, provide direction. Is the patient able to communicate verbally, by writing, or texting? Are assistive devices needed? Ask the patient and family about preferences for meeting, considering timing, location, and privacy needs. If a family member is distraught, providing a quiet place away from the bedside might facilitate open expression. If the patient can participate, plan to hold the meeting when the patient is rested and when his or her pain is well-managed, to promote optimal participation. Discussions concerning ethical issues and conflicts in care are complex and should be held in the language most comfortable for the patient and family. If English is not the preferred language for health care conversations, provide a trained medical interpreter for the meetings. Be present for individual meetings with the patient and family unless contraindicated for a specific reason.

Participate in the Consultation Meeting

Any ethics consultation meeting concerning an inpatient should have a representative of the nursing staff at the table. If a nurse initiated the consult, ideally this nurse should participate in the meeting. First, the nurse's perspective on the experience and burden of care is essential. Also, as various treatment options are discussed, the nurse can provide reality testing. Proposed clinical interventions might not be possible in reality. Nurses can address available resources and solve problems to ensure treatment options under consideration are implementable. The bedside nurses' concerns and perspectives on the care issues should be visible. Given schedules and care demands, nurses might identify a particular nurse to represent this perspective in the discussion. Although managers might also need and want to participate, the involvement of the bedside nurse is recommended.

Difficult health care decisions carry a heavy moral burden for the clinicians who must act upon them. Witnessing suffering, caring for actively dying patients, and being present with those who grieve are moral obligations of bedside nurses. With these obligations comes the right to be part of the process that informs decisions and drives the care that nurses provide.

Learn from the Consultation Process

A variety of methodologies and processes exist for clinical ethics consultations (ASBH, 2009). Consultants vary in academic preparation and clinical experience, but in general, the consultant engages in ethical analysis and facilitates moral deliberations about the ethically justifiable options. "An effective consultation process creates deliberate opportunities to seek the perspective of all the involved parties, anticipating and even expecting that they may frame the issues and questions differently and may have different and competing perspectives" (ASBH, 2009, p. 63.). The outcomes from the consultation process vary and might include identifying the ethically appropriate decision-maker, distinguishing numerous treatment options that can be ethically justifiable, or supporting the patient's right to reject or receive life-sustaining treatment. Most consultants document in the medical record and provide references and background ethics literature to facilitate understanding of the consult's outcomes. After the consultation is documented, some consultants continue to follow the patient's care and provide support for the team.

Nurses requesting or participating in an ethics consultation can expect to learn from the process. Ethics committees and consultants generally consider ethics education an important aspect of their work. Review the consult note in the chart. If some aspect of the process is confusing, seek clarification. Ask the consultant for relevant articles from the ethics literature. The consultant can offer supporting literature and identify relevant professional codes, organizational policies, and pieces of legislation that have informed the consultation. The *Code of Medical Ethics* of the American Medical Association often provides relevant opinions on issues that trouble nurses. The American Nurses Association issues position statements on many aspects of care, including, for example, forgoing nutrition and hydration.

Recognize that decisions for a patient's care are not made by an ethics consultant. Authority for care remains with the patient or his or her legally authorized surrogate decision-maker in collaboration with the clinicians providing care. Although nurses and physicians might find that the consultation outcomes do not represent their personal values, ideally they will at least understand the ethical analysis and the need to honor the patient's preference and values.

Identify Issues for Follow-Up

Talk with nursing leadership after a complex patient care situation. Would a gathering of the staff to discuss feelings and concerns be beneficial? Is a nurse ethicist available to discuss recurring practice patterns that raise moral concerns for the staff? Is a pattern to the ethics consultations emerging in a specific unit or specialty practice? Are nurses experiencing moral distress? Identify nurses in the work group who have an interest in ethics, and consider approaches to making ethical questions and concerns visible and routine areas of discussion. Could a standard prompt be added to the change of shift report and rounds to elicit potential ethical concerns?

Conclusion

Certain patients, their loved ones, and the experiences of caring for them remain with us. They might even haunt us after troubling ethics consultations (Ford & Dudzinski, 2008). What was the right thing to do, and what made it so? These experiences of care embedded with moral concerns shape nursing identities and practice. They inform the care we will provide to future patients and their families. "Nursing care aims to maximize the values that the patient has treasured in life and extends supportive care to the family and significant others" (ANA, 2001, p. 7). Ethics consultation is an effective resource to assist nursing in achieving these aims.

Talk About It!

- Start a conversation with your colleagues about the values expressed in your work setting. Think in terms of personal values, professional values, and specialty practice values. Explore experiences from other practice settings. Do they differ from your current one?

- Consider the values of aggressive care to generate new knowledge and skills and then contrast with the concept of "the good death." How do you feel about finding a balance?

- Identify areas where the approach to care differs—perhaps in regard to management of pain or engaging family members in direct patient-care activities. Explore ways to launch a discussion that invites a variety of beliefs and opinions to be expressed. Did the discussion evolve to identify and consider the range of values? Are there any hidden values in your group or organization? Did some colleagues feel the need to defend their own values? If so, how might you reshape the conversation to promote open discussion?

- Find out about the membership of your practice setting's ethics committee. Contact a representation and discuss some of the ethical concerns that prompt consultation. Is there a nurse member of the committee or on the consult service? Ask your colleagues about any experiences with ethics consultation. Was the experience valuable? Who sought the consult? What did they learn from the experience? Would they call a consult in the future based on their past experience?

- Identify a value or belief that one of your patients or their family members expressed that made you think about your own values related to the issue. Would you feel comfortable asking your patient questions to gain a greater understanding of their value or belief? Would you be inclined to ask more questions or want to offer your alternate opinion? Would this vary if it were spiritual belief, in contrast to a health care belief, that's inconsistent with your beliefs? Practice sharing the belief with a colleague without conveying your opinion. Was it difficult to hold back your opinion?

References

American Association of Critical-Care Nurses. (2011). *Beacon award for excellence application handbook.* Retrieved from http://www.aacn.org/wd/beaconapps/content/mainpage.pcms?menu=beaconapps

American Nurses Association. (2001). *Code of ethics for nurses with interpretive statements.* Washington, DC: Author.

American Nurses Association. (2008). *Guide to the code of ethics for nurses: Interpretation and application.* M.D.M. Fowler (Ed.). Silver Spring, MD: Author.

American Nurses Association. (2010). *Nursing's social policy statement: The essence of the profession.* Silver Spring, MD: Author.

American Nurses Credentialing Center. (2008). *Magnet recognition program: Application manual 2008.* Silver Spring, MD: Author.

American Society for Bioethics and Humanities. (2009). *Improving competencies in clinical ethics consultations: An education guide.* Glenview, IL: Author.

American Society for Bioethics and Humanities. (2011). *Core competencies for healthcare ethics consultation* (3rd ed.). Glenview, IL: Author.

Aulisio, M. P., & Arnold, R. M. (2008). Role of the ethics committee: Helping to address value conflicts or uncertainties. *Chest, 134*(2), 417-424.

Bu, Z., & Jezewski, M. A. (2006). Developing a mid-range theory of patient advocacy through concept analysis. *Journal of Advanced Nursing, 57*(1), 101-110. doi:10.1111/j.1365-2648.2006.04096.x

Craig, J. M., & May, T. (2006). Evaluating the outcomes of ethics consultation. *The Journal of Clinical Ethics, 17*(2), 168-180.

Danis, M., Farrar, A., Grady, C., Taylor, C., O'Donnell, P., Soekem, K., & Ulrich, C. (2008). Does fear of retaliation deter request for ethics consultation. *Medicine, Health Care and Philosophy: A European Journal, 11,* 27-34.

DeWolf Bosek, M. S. (2009). Identifying ethical issues from the perspective of the registered nurse. *JONA's Healthcare Law, Ethics, and Regulation, 11*(3), 91-99.

Dubler, N. N., Webber, M. P., Swiderski, D. M., & the Faculty and the National Working Group for the Clinical Ethics Credentialing Project. (2009). Charting the future: Credentialing, privileging, quality, and evaluation in clinical ethics consultation. *Hastings Center Report, 39*(6), 23-33.

Ethics Resource Center. (2009, May 29). *Definitions of values.* Retrieved from http://www.ethics.org/resource/definitions-values

Ford, P. J., & Dudzinski, D. M. (2008). *Complex ethics consultations: Cases that haunt us.* New York: Cambridge University Press.

Fox, E., Berkowitz, K. A., Chanko, B. L., & Powell, T. (2006). *Ethics consultation: Responding to ethics question in health care.* Washington, DC: Veterans Health Administration. Retrieved from http//:www.ethics.va.gov/docs/integratedethics/Ethics_Consultation_Responding_to_Ethics_Questions_in_Health_Care_20070808.pdf

Fox, E., Myers, S., & Pearlman R. A. (2007). Ethics consultation in United States hospitals: A national survey. *American Journal of Bioethics, 7*(2), 13-25.

Gentile, M. C. (2010). *Giving voice to values: How to speak your mind when you know what's right.* New Haven, CT: Yale University Press.

Gordon, E. J., & Hamric, A. B. (2006). The courage to stand up: The cultural politics of nurses' access to ethics consultation. *The Journal of Clinical Ethics, 17*(3), 231-254.

Hamric, A. B. (2000). What is happening to advocacy? *Nursing Outlook, 48*(3), 103-104.

Hamric, A. B. (2001). Reflections on being in the middle. *Nursing Outlook, 49*(6), 254-257.

The Joint Commission. (2011). *The comprehensive accreditation manual for hospitals (CAMH) and homecare (CAMH).* Oakbrook, IL: Author.

Murphy, P. (1993). Clinical ethics: Must nurses be forever in the middle? *Bioethics Forum, 9*(4), 3-4.

Varcoe, C., Doane, G., Pauly, B., Rodney, P., Storch, J. L., Mahoney, K.,… Starzomski, R. (2004). Ethical practice in nursing: Working the in-betweens. *Journal of Advanced Nursing, 45*(3), 316-325.

GENETICS AND GENOMICS IN THE 21ST CENTURY: ETHICAL CONSIDERATIONS

–Kathleen A. Calzone, PhD, RN, APNG, FAAN
Senior Nurse Specialist, Research
National Institutes of Health, National Cancer Institute
Center for Cancer Research, Genetics Branch

6

Think About It!

Genetic and genomic information and technology:

- Can be collected, analyzed, and stored prior to conception, at any point in a person's life, and after death.

- Predict future health risks, but prediction is not absolute and results can also be unexpected or incidental findings (i.e., misattributed paternity).

- Create an opportunity for misinterpretation or misuse.

- Alter lifestyle, family relationships, reproductive decision-making, and health behaviors (i.e., increased screening or risk-reducing surgery).

- Nurses are optimally positioned to contribute to the ethical translation of genetic and genomic information and technology into health care.

Genetic/genomic information is already being used to identify people and families at risk for certain conditions, better inform screening and risk-reduction options, screen for certain conditions, inform prognostic and therapeutic decisions, develop targeted therapies, and personalize therapy by informing medication selection and dosing. These advancing technologies and this knowledge about genetics and genomics influence the entire wellness-to-illness health care continuum and, therefore, are fundamental to all nursing practice (Calzone, et al., 2010). Though initially many of the discoveries were not ready for clinical application, the rapidity in which these discoveries are transitioning to the clinical arena has accelerated (Feero, Guttmacher, & Collins, 2010). And though advances in genetics/genomics also have significant potential to improve health outcomes, they also present a myriad of ethical challenges.

> ### Case Study 6.1
>
> Maria is a healthy female, 39, married for 15 years, a vegetarian, a marathon runner, an avid exerciser, with a good body weight (low BMI), and is an information seeker. She has a teenage boy and a preteen girl, both living with her and her husband. They live in a large city, downtown. Maria works at a very stressful job as an accountant and is very computer literate. She does not have a routine primary care provider because she is otherwise healthy. She presents to a local family practice as a new patient, because she has had a full genome scan performed by a direct-to-consumer testing company, and results revealed an increased risk of cardiovascular disease and heart attack. She feels she is doomed to have a heart attack and has been emotionally distraught by this information. She did not expect to learn information that would impact her long-term health, even though she knew that this was a possibility.

Genetics refers to the study of individual genes associated with rare single gene disorders that are often rare in the general population, whereas *genomics* refers to the study of the entire human genome and other influencing variables including personal, environmental, psychosocial, and cultural (Guttmacher & Collins, 2002). In fact, even in the setting of a single gene disorder, those genes are not operating in isolation, but continue to interface with other genes and the other factors just listed. Therefore, the term *genomics* encompasses the current state of the science and is the term used throughout this chapter.

What is genomic information? Is it only generated as a result of a genetic test? No, genomic information can be collected without ever collecting a biospecimen. Encounters with a health care provider are one of the most common mechanisms for collecting genomic information. How many of you have even collected your own or a patient's family health history? If you have, then you have collected genomic information, and you could argue that you have just performed the cheapest and most widely accessible genomic test there is. Many non-biospecimen-related sources of genomic information exist. These can include physical features that are common in biologic family members. Think about the large nose that runs in the family, or a physical trait or disease that when present indicates a genetic disorder, such as cystic fibrosis. These are also sources of genomic information. Only recently has the collection of a biospecimen been an increasingly common source of genomic information.

In the current environment, you can find something almost daily in the lay medial or professional literature related to DNA and/or genomics. In health care, new developments occur regularly, so why all the fuss? Is genomics different from other health information and technology? Probably not as much as you might think. However, there are some important considerations concerning this information. Genomic information can:

- Be gathered, stored, and analyzed at any point from preconception to after death
- Alter lifestyle choices, such as reproductive decision-making
- Have implications for biological family members and influence family relationships
- Influence a person's physical, intellectual, and emotional attributes and traits
- Create opportunities for misuse
- Provide information about future health risks in otherwise healthy individuals
- Reveal unexpected findings (such as misattributed paternity)

- Raise questions about the distinction among risks, traits, and disease

- Reveal your personal identity

These considerations should not lead to genomic exceptionalism, the idea that genomic information is somehow different from any other health information (Evans, Burke, & Khoury, 2010). In fact, if you think about it, many types of health information can result in similar effects. Consider some of these examples. Could being diagnosed with cancer as a young adult influence reproductive decisions? Can developing an infectious disease impact biologic family members? Could a biopsy that reveals abnormal cells such as atypical hyperplasia of the breast provide information about future health risks? The answer to all these questions is yes.

So, what is unique about genomic information? The ability to use DNA, in even very small amounts, to reveal your personal identity. DNA is the ultimate identifier. In addition, you can learn genomic information about a person before they are born and long after they have died. Another distinction is that genomics is a science that, though not new, is one in which most health care providers have had little to no preparation. Studies of health care professionals worldwide over the last several years indicate very little improvement in genomic knowledge, despite education efforts. Therefore, most health care providers are not sufficiently competent in genomics to understand this information and integrate this into their practice. For the benefits of genomics to reach the patient, health care providers, including nurses, must be knowledgeable about the influence of this information and technology on health care and have sufficient command of the information to integrate this information ethically and appropriately into their practice (Consensus Panel on Genetic/Genomic Nursing Competencies, 2009). With the rapid expansion of clinically relevant genomic information, the preparation of the health care workforce in ethically informed genomics is a priority. This chapter provides an overview of the ethical challenges associated with translating genomic discoveries into practice and provides resources to help you learn even more.

Genetic Testing

Though genomic information can be collected just as part of routine health care, when should health care providers consider doing an actual genetic test? In today's technology- and information-driven society, shouldn't we do testing if it is available? Isn't more information better? Not necessarily. What if you can't interpret the results of the test? Or, what if the test you perform will not give you any additional information that could help in the diagnosis or treatment of a given condition? Or, what if the personal or family history is not suggestive for the condition you might do testing for (American Society of Clinical Oncology, 2003; Robson, Storm, Weitzel, Wollins, & Offit, 2010)? In addition, many of these tests can be very expensive, so careful consideration of when to consider testing is essential.

Will testing always be so expensive? No. This is one area of health care that has already seen dramatic reductions in cost. Continued developments in technology have enabled DNA sequencing to be done quicker and at a decreased price (Pettersson, Lundeberg, & Ahmadian, 2009; Snyder, Jiang Du, & Gerstein, 2010). In fact, we are on the precipice of the $1,000 genome, which refers to the ability to sequence someone's entire genome for $1,000. Though not yet available, experts agree this will happen in the near future; it is just a matter of when (National Human Genome Research Institute, 2010).

How will the $1,000 genome be applied in health care? The potential applications span the entire health care continuum from preconception to end of life and beyond. Yet, the challenge of how health care providers can harness this information to optimize health care remains to be determined. However, genomic health care applications already are being translated into practice and will only accelerate with further potential to expand newborn screening, identify at-risk individuals, diagnose health conditions, and personalize health care and treatment.

Case Study (cont.)

Maria's mother was Puerto Rican and died when she was 35 and Maria was very young. Her father refuses to talk about what happened, because she was in a motor vehicle accident and he was driving the car and survived without any injury. Maria doesn't know much about her mother or her family, but in pictures she is Caucasian. However, Maria's father won't provide any details. Maria knows her mother grew up in Puerto Rico, but doesn't know if she was really Puerto Rican by blood. She decided to have genetic testing to learn more about her ethnic heritage, especially from her mother's side of the family. However, the health information was something she never expected.

Direct-to-Consumer Testing

One of the most interesting trends in genetic testing had been the advent of direct-to-consumer (DTC) marketing or testing. Certainly direct-to-consumer marketing of pharmaceuticals and medical devices is commonplace. But the ability to order your own genetic test is a novel development. Interest and uptake of DTC testing are not well known at this time. However evidence is emerging that consumers of DTC testing are at risk of misinterpreting the findings (Leighton, Valverde, & Bernhardt, 2011). The availability of these tests continues to expand and encompass testing for risks of common health conditions such as cancer and cardiovascular disease, ancestry, common personal traits, pharmacogenomics, and nutrition (Genetics and Public Policy Center, 2011). Availability of DTC tests does not equate to clinical validity, the likelihood that a given genetic variant is associated with a specific utility, or the value of the test in improving health outcomes (Haddow & Palomaki, 2003).

Case Study (cont.)

Maria has two children, a son who is 13 years old and a daughter who is 10. Both are in good health and in school. She hasn't talked with them about this but really wants them to be tested, because she wants to know if she passed this risk for cardiovascular disease on to her children.

Testing in Children and Vulnerable Populations

For the purposes of genetic testing, children are considered anyone younger than 18 years of age. When should genetic testing be considered in children? As illustrated by the continuing case study throughout this chapter and the current evidence, parents often are very interested in testing their children even for adult-onset conditions for which no known risks or changes in medical management would occur before legal adulthood (Bradbury et al., 2010; Tercyak et al., 2011). However, experts in genomics feel that testing should be deferred until adulthood unless the test will change medical management (American Society of Clinical Oncology, 2003; American Society of Human Genetics Board of Directors, 1995). This recommendation is in part related to concerns about psychological and developmental impacts. However, for a number of genetic disorders, testing is recommended in children because health implications exist for those children. These can include disorders such as familial hypercholesterolemia, cystic fibrosis, or fragile X as well as cancer syndromes such as retinoblastoma or multiple endocrine neoplasia (MEN) types 1 and 2 (Tischkowitz & Rosser, 2004; Wertz, Fanos, & Reilly, 1994).

Genetic education, counseling, and testing in children present some important aspects to consider. A child's age and developmental stage can influence the degree in which a child is involved in the genetic testing decision. For example, children over age 10 might have more involvement versus younger children. The important variable is not a child's precise age, as children develop differently, but whether the child is at a developmental stage to understand the genetic testing process, the results, and the associated health implications (Fanos, 1997). Regardless of age, a parent or legal representative must be involved in the decision-making and consent to test. Genetic testing can affect emotional development, parent/child bonding, and degree of anxiety, or result in guilt, and the risk might not be understood (Fanos, 1997).

In summary, if genetic testing in a child is being considered, a careful assessment of developmental stage is needed to determine the degree to which the child is involved in the testing decision. In addition, the genetic counseling needs to address the potential psychosocial and cognitive outcomes of testing. In young children, how test results will be shared when the child is older needs to be addressed (American Society of Clinical Oncology, 2003). Lastly, evidence that the test would alter health care is important when considering whether to offer testing to children.

Vulnerable populations are another group that necessitates special considerations with genetic testing. The definition of a vulnerable population varies. The International Society of Nurses in Genetics (ISONG) adopted the broadest definition, encompassing the 45 CFR Code of Federal Regulations part 46 Protection Of Human Subjects, which includes children, pregnant women, prisoners, patients who are traumatized, comatose patients, terminally ill, disabled, or cognitively impaired (Department of Health and Human Services, 2009) as well as other variables that ISONG felt constituted vulnerability, including hearing, language, or communication impairments and psychosocial variables, such as psychiatric conditions, stress, or financial issues (International Society of Nurses in Genetics, 2010).

ISONG's position is that genetic testing in vulnerable populations includes an assessment of physical, cognitive and developmental stages; genetic literacy; and interest in genomics, and establishes outcomes in partnership with the interdisciplinary health care team that are consistent with the individual's goals (International Society of Nurses in Genetics, 2010). As is the case with testing in children, a legal representative such as a durable power of attorney might be required to consent for genetic testing.

Evaluating Genetic Tests

How do you then evaluate genetic tests? The Centers for Disease Control and Prevention has developed the ACCE model (Figure 6.1), which stands for **a**nalytic validity; **c**linical validity; **c**linical utility; and **e**thical, legal, and social implications (Office of Surveillance, 2010). Analytic validity refers to the tests' ability to accurately assess a given genotype. Clinical validity is the likelihood that the specific genotype is associated with a given health condition. Clinical utility refers to the likelihood that results of a specific genetic test can improve health outomces. The ACCE model provides a series of 44 specific questions that can help providers evaluate genetic tests (Office of Surveillance, 2010). Current discussions propose expanding this model to also consider personal utility, public utility, and economic value (Foster, Mulvihill, & Sharp, 2009; Institute of Medicine Roundtable on Translating Genomic-Based Research for Health, 2010).

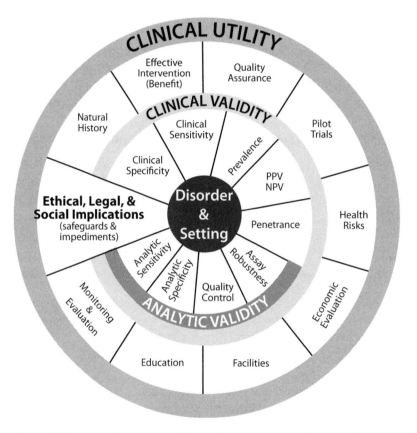

Figure 6.1 ACCE Model (analytic validity; clinical validity; clinical utility; and ethical, legal and, social implications) for assessing genetic tests (Haddow & Palomaki, 2003).

Case Study (cont.)

Maria has a half-sister who is part American Indian and lives on an Indian reservation in Arizona. She also has two children but does not have the financial resources needed to pay for this testing. Maria has decided to offer her the testing as a gift. However, Maria's half-sister obtains her health care through the Indian Health Service and is unsure whether someone there can answer her questions, because she is in such a rural area. In addition, Maria's half-sister is aware of the tribal sensitivities associated with genetic/genomic information and, as a consequence, has personal and tribal beliefs that influence her interest in this testing. Though she is interested in this testing if it could benefit her children, she is feeling pressured to get testing by her sister Maria.

Genomic Health Care Equality

As genetic testing becomes more pervasive, this raises the concern that access to genetic/genomic tests is predominately limited to individuals with insurance coverage or the ability to pay (Calzone et al., 2010). Access to genetic services is not only about finances but also encompasses access for racial, ethnic, and cultural minorities as well as those in geographically isolated areas (Hawkins & Hayden, 2011). To address some of the geographic isolation, some regions of the country are developing regional service programs, whereas other genetic services are offering outreach programs. Table 6.1 lists some of the resources available for finding a genetic health care professional. If no one is in the area you seek, consider contacting the closest provider to investigate whether regional or outreach genetic services are available.

Table 6.1   Find a Genetic Health Care Professional

Resource	Location
American Society of Human Genetics	http://www.ashg.org/
International Society of Nurses in Genetics	http://www.isong.org/
National Society of Genetic Counselors, Find a Genetic Counselor	http://www.nsgc.org/tabid/69/Default.aspx
National Cancer Institute Cancer Genetics Services Directory	http://www.cancer.gov/cancertopics/genetics/directory

Genetic Education and Counseling

At the heart of genetic education and counseling is the goal of autonomous, informed decision-making regarding genetic testing to facilitate optimal understanding of the result and adjustment to the health implications (Elwyn, Gray, & Clarke, 2000). The National Society of Genetic Counselors has defined genetic counseling as "the process of helping people understand and adapt to the medical, psychological, and familial implications of genetic contributions to disease. This process integrates the following:

- Interpretation of family and medical histories to assess the chance of disease occurrence or recurrence

- Education about inheritance, testing, management, prevention, resources, and research

- Counseling to promote informed choices and adaptation to the risk or condition" (National Society of Genetic Counselors' Definition Task Force, 2006).

Genetic counseling can be delivered by a number of methods, such as traditional in-person encounters, group education followed by individual encounters, computer-assisted counseling, and telegenomics, which is the use of telemedicine services for genetic counseling (Calzone et al., 2005; Green, Biesecker, McInerney, Mauger, & Fost, 2001; Stalker et al., 2006).

Most experts agree that genetic testing should not be performed without genetic counseling by a trained health care professional. Who is qualified to deliver genetic/genomic services? Several types of providers have specialty training in genomics, and they include:

- Medical geneticists who are certified by the American Board of Medical Genetics

- Genetic counselors who are certified by the American Board of Genetic Counseling or American Board of Medical Genetics

- Genetic nurses who are credentialed by the Genetic Nursing Credentialing Commission

Refer back to Table 6.1 for a list of some of the resources available for finding a genetic health care professional.

Psychosocial Issues

Genomics can result in psychological issues not only for the individual, but also for the family. In general, many studies have demonstrated that genetic testing does not result in adverse psychological outcomes, and most people will adapt well to the information (Broadstock, Michie, & Marteau, 2000; Meiser, 2005). However, not everyone will do well regardless of their test result. Risk factors for distress following genetic testing include those with a personal history of depression, those with elevated distress prior to undergoing genetic testing, those who obtain an unexpected result, those who have results that differ from siblings, those with ongoing problems with the condition in the family, and individuals with small children (Meiser, 2005). These risk factors point to the need for critical assessments performed prior to genetic testing to help identify those individuals who might develop problems following testing and to allow for interventions to reduce that risk. Interventions to consider when encountering a high-risk individual include involvement of a mental health professional early in the genetic education, counseling, and testing process.

Genomics is a family affair, and though a test might be suggested for a specific family member, inherited conditions have implications for other biologic family members. A particular issue is that of who is the most informative person to test first in a family. For conditions transmitted in an autosomal dominant fashion (only one copy of the disease-associated mutation is needed to cause the health condition), testing a family member who already is affected with the condition is most informative. Testing an unaffected family member without knowing the specific gene and mutation associated with a health condition in the family can result in a false negative. No mutation detected could be because the individual has not inherited the family mutation, but also could be because the family has no identifiable mutation in the tested gene, in which case the individual is still at an increased risk for that condition. In the absence of a known mutation in the family, no genetic testing technique has 100% sensitivity, nor are all of the genes and gene modifiers associated with certain health conditions discovered.

One result of this conundrum is that someone who can benefit most from the test might be advised to have another family member tested first who would be more informative. This can result in instances of family coercion, especially difficult when a family member decides he or she does not want to know this information. Though this sounds manageable by educating and counseling the individual interested in testing on the limitations of a negative result, the right of a family member not to know can be jeopardized. Consider the case of an obligate carrier (Figure 6.2). Individual A is interested in genetic testing for the mutation that has been found in her maternal aunt, individual D. However, individual C, the patient's mother, has decided she does not want to be tested, because she does not want to know this information. If the mutation in the maternal aunt, individual D, is found in our patient, individual A, then her mother, individual C, must have passed the family mutation to her. So, the results of the mother can actually be determined even if the mother has decided she does not want to know. Education and counseling addressing the impact of this circumstance are essential prior to initiating any testing.

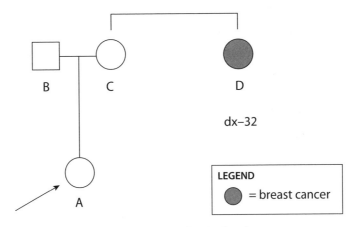

Figure 6.2 Obligate Carrier

Because genomics has implications for biologic family members, the assessment extends beyond the individual to include the family as well. Assessments include patterns of communication, family management of the cancer history to date, patterns of health care decision-making within the family, roles and relationships within the family, and cultural and family beliefs that might influence health care (Miller, McDaniel, Rolland, & Feetham, 2006). Keep in mind, an individual might consider people who are important to the family social system as family members, even if they are not biologically related, and these individuals can be important in health care decision-making (Olsen, Dudley-Brown, & McMullen, 2004).

Outcomes of genetic testing for the family can spark a range of responses. For example, if a gene mutation is identified, this result could engender different types of guilt: transmitter guilt experienced by parents who learn they passed a gene mutation on to their children or survivor guilt in a family member who is not found to have the gene mutation affecting the other family members. Pre- and post-test genetic education and counseling are intended to help families anticipate outcomes, prepare for these responses, and help them adapt to their results.

The outcomes of genetic testing are also important for biologic family members who might be at risk for having the same gene mutation associated with the health condition(s). Who is told, how, and how accurate family communication of genomic information is remain a source of important study. Work done to date has shown that sharing this information within the family might be limited to those who are closely related, such as first- or second-degree relatives. When to tell and how to tell children varies, and those of the gender affected by the health condition, such as women and breast cancer, might be told more than members of the opposite gender (Ersig, Hadley, & Koehly, 2011; Hughes et al., 2002; Metcalfe, Coad, Plumridge, Gill, & Farndon, 2008).

Case Study (cont.)

Maria is asked by the family practice health care provider for a copy of her genetic testing report for her medical record. Maria is concerned about whether the information about her risk for cardiovascular disease could be used to discriminate against her.

Privacy and Confidentiality

Genomic information derived from clinical data, such as symptoms of an illness or family history or the results of a genetic test, raises the risk of discrimination for the individuals and their family for employment or different types of insurance discrimination (Klitzman, 2010). Laws at both the state and federal level have been passed that help to address some concerns of employment and health insurance discrimination. However, protections against life, long-term care, and disability insurances are limited.

The most notable development in the protections against discrimination was the passage of the Genetic Information Nondiscrimination Act (GINA) in 2008. This federal legislation applies to health insurance and employment discrimination based on genetic information. This law provides a minimum amount of protection but does not supersede more extensive protections provided by a given state. GINA prevents insurers from:

- Accessing a person's genetic information

- Requiring an individual to undergo any kind of genetic test

- Using genomic information against a person during medical underwriting

GINA still allows for someone's current health status to be considered during medical underwriting for health insurance. Coverage for tests and procedures is not influenced by GINA. In addition, GINA does not alter a health care provider's access to an individual's genomic information (Genetics and Public Policy Center, 2008; National Cancer Institute PDQ Genetics Editorial Board, 2011).

GINA prevents employers from:

- Accessing a person's genetic information

- Using genomic information to deny employment

- Collecting genetic or genomic information without explicit consent

Employment agencies and labor organizations also cannot use genomic information to determine whether or not to refer an individual for employment. In addition, labor organizations cannot use genomic information in membership decisions. Employers are still allowed to perform occupational testing for toxic substances (Genetics and Public Policy Center, 2008; National Cancer Institute PDQ Genetics Editorial Board, 2011).

GINA protections do not provide provisions for life, long-term care, or disability insurances. The protections provided by GINA also do not extend to active duty military personnel, the Veterans Benefits

Administration, or the Indian Health Service. These coverage gaps exist because existing laws were amended through GINA, and those laws do not apply to these programs or services (Baruch & Hudson, 2008; National Cancer Institute PDQ Genetics Editorial Board, 2011).

The National Human Genome Research Institute (NHGRI) maintains a website at http://www.genome.gov/10002077 on genetic discrimination that provides an overview of all the considerations related to discrimination on the basis of genetic or genomic information. NHGRI also maintains a Genome Statute and Legislative Database (see website link in Table 6.2), which provides summaries of statutes and bills that address privacy, employment, and insurance discrimination from 2007 onward. The National Cancer Institute PDQ Cancer Genetics Risk Assessment and Counseling summary at http://www.cancer.gov/cancertopics/pdq/genetics/risk-assessment-and-counseling/HealthProfessional/page6#Section_386 maintains an overview of the landscape of federal and state protections against insurance and employment discrimination.

Table 6.2   Selected Resources on Ethical Issues and Genomics

Resource	Location
Centers for Disease Control and Prevention National Office of Public Health Genomics	http://www.cdc.gov/genomics/
Coalition for Genetic Fairness	http://www.geneticfairness.org/
Council for Responsible Genetics	http://www.gene-watch.org
Genetic Alliance	http://www.geneticalliance.org/
Genetics and Ethics in Health Care: New Questions in the Age of Genomic Health Editor: Rita Black Monsen	American Nurses Association http://www.nursesbooks.org/Main-Menu/Ethics/Genetics-and-Ethics-In-Health-Care.aspx
Genetics & Public Policy Center	http://www.dnapolicy.org/
Genome Statute and Legislative Database	http://www.genome.gov/PolicyEthics/LegDatabase/pubsearch.cfm
National Institutes of Health Bioethics Resources on the Web	http://bioethics.od.nih.gov/
Secretary's Advisory Committee on Genetics, Health, & Society	http://oba.od.nih.gov/SACGHS/sacghs_home.html
Your Genes, Your Choices	http://www.ornl.gov/sci/techresources/Human_Genome/publicat/genechoice/index.html

Conclusion

Professional guidelines and other resources (refer back to Table 6.2) exist to help nurses and other health professionals understand more about some of the ethical issues and options available as more genomics information is translated into clinical care. In addition, consultation with genetic health care professionals (refer back to Table 6.1) can be of value when a potential ethical issue is recognized and either you or your local resources could benefit from additional consultation. This is an exciting time to be in health care, where the use of genetic/genomic information and technology is transforming health care into a truly personalized approach. Nurses especially are well-positioned to help patients, because they are the most trusted health care providers, the ones who can truly facilitate the ethical translation of genomics to improve patient care (Calzone et al., 2010).

Talk About It!

- How are you using genomic information in your nursing practice today? What changes in your practice would you expect as more genomic information is translated into health care? Talk to your colleagues about the scope of genomic information used in your practice environment and the current and future impact on nursing practice.

- Do you know who and how to reach genetic health care providers in your area for consultation or referral? Consider identifying your local genetic health care provider resources.

- How prepared are you to answer your patients' questions about genomics? What can you do to ensure you and your colleagues are competent in genomics?

References

American Society of Clinical Oncology. (2003). American Society of Clinical Oncology policy statement update: Genetic testing for cancer susceptibility. *Journal of Clinical Oncology, 21*(12), 2397-2406.

American Society of Human Genetics Board of Directors, A. C. o. M. G. B. o. D. (1995). Points to consider: Ethical, legal, and psychosocial implications of genetic testing in children and adolescents. *American Journal of Human Genetics, 57*(5), 1233-1241.

Baruch, S., & Hudson, K. (2008). Civilian and military genetics: Nondiscrimination policy in a post-GINA world. *American Journal of Human Genetics, 83*(4), 435-444.

Bradbury, A. R., Patrick-Miller, L., Egleston, B., Sands, C. B., Li, T., Schmidheiser, H., … Daugherty, C. K. (2010). Parent opinions regarding the genetic testing of minors for BRCA1/2. *Journal of Clinical Oncology, 28*(21), 3498-3505.

Broadstock, M., Michie, S., & Marteau, T. (2000). Psychological consequences of predictive genetic testing: A systematic review. *European Journal of Human Genetics, 8*(10), 731-738.

Calzone, K. A., Cashion, A., Feetham, S., Jenkins, J., Prows, C. A., Williams, J. K., & Wung, S. F. (2010). Nurses transforming health care using genetics and genomics. *Nursing Outlook, 58*(1), 26-35.

Calzone, K. A., Prindiville, S. A., Jourkiv, O., Jenkins, J., DeCarvalho, M., Wallerstedt, D. B., … Kirsch, I. R. (2005). A randomized comparison of group versus individual genetic education and counseling for familial breast and/or ovarian cancer. *Journal of Clinical Oncology, 23*, 3455-3464.

Consensus Panel on Genetic/Genomic Nursing Competencies. (2009). *Essentials of genetic and genomic nursing: Competencies, curricula guidelines, and outcome indicators* (2nd ed.). Silver Spring, MD: American Nurses Association.

Department of Health and Human Services. (2009). *Code of federal regulations, title 45, public welfare, part 46, protection of human subjects*. Washington, DC: Department of Health and Human Services. Retrieved from http://www.hhs.gov/ohrp/policy/ohrpregulations.pdf

Elwyn, G., Gray, J., & Clarke, A. (2000). Shared decision making and non-directiveness in genetic counselling. *Journal of Medical Genetics, 37*(2), 135-138.

Ersig, A. L., Hadley, D. W., & Koehly, L. M. (2011). Understanding patterns of health communication in families at risk for hereditary nonpolyposis colorectal cancer: Examining the effect of conclusive versus indeterminate genetic test results. *Health Communication, 26*(7), 587-594.

Evans, J. P., Burke, W., Khoury, M. (2010). The rules remain the same for genomic medicine: The case against "reverse genetic exceptionalism". *Genetics in Medicine, 12*(6), 342-343.

Fanos, J. H. (1997). Developmental tasks of childhood and adolescence: Implications for genetic testing. *American Journal of Medical Genetics, 71*(1), 22-28.

Feero, W. G., Guttmacher, A. E., & Collins, F. S. (2010). Genomic medicine--An updated primer. *New England Journal of Medicine, 362*(21), 2001-2011.

Foster, M. W., Mulvihill, J. J., & Sharp, R. R. (2009). Evaluating the utility of personal genomic information. *Genetics in Medicine, 11*(8), 570-574.

Genetics and Public Policy Center. (2008). *Information on the Genetic Information Nondiscrimination Act (GINA)*. Retrieved from http://www.dnapolicy.org/resources/WhatGINAdoesanddoesnotdochart.pdf

Genetics and Public Policy Center. (2011). *DTC genetic testing companies.* Retrieved from http://www.dnapolicy.org/resources/DTCAug2011byDiseasecategory.pdf

Green, M. J., Biesecker, B. B., McInerney, A. M., Mauger, D., & Fost, N. (2001). An interactive computer program can effectively educate patients about genetic testing for breast cancer susceptibility. *American Journal of Medical Genetics, 103*(1), 16-23.

Guttmacher, A., & Collins, F. S. (2002). Genomic medicine: A primer. *New England Journal of Medicine, 347*, 1512-1520.

Haddow, J. E., & Palomaki, G. E. (2003). ACCE: A model process for evaluating data on emerging genetic tests. In M. Khoury, J. Little, & W. Burke (Eds.). *Human genome epidemiology: A scientific foundation for using genetic information to improve health and prevent disease* (pp. 217-233). New York: Oxford University Press.

Hawkins, A. K., & Hayden, M. R. (2011). A grand challenge: Providing benefits of clinical genetics to those in need. *Genetics in Medicine, 13*(3), 197-200.

Hughes, C., Lerman, C., Schwartz, M., Peshkin, B. N., Wenzel, L., Narod, S., … Main, D. (2002). All in the family: Evaluation of the process and content of sisters' communication about BRCA1 and BRCA2 genetic test results. *American Journal of Medical Genetics, 107*(2), 143-150.

Institute of Medicine Roundtable on Translating Genomic-Based Research for Health. (2010). *The value of genetic and genomic technologies: Workshop summary.* Washington DC: National Academies Press.

International Society of Nurses in Genetics. (2010). *Genetic counseling for vulnerable populations: The role of nursing.* Retrieved from http://www.isong.org/ISONG_PS_genetic_counseling_vulnerable_populations.php

Klitzman, R. (2010). Views of discrimination among individuals confronting genetic disease. *Journal of Genetic Counseling, 19*(1), 68-83.

Leighton, J. W., Valverde, K., & Bernhardt, B. A. (2011). The general public's understanding and perception of direct-to-consumer genetic test results. *Public Health Genomics, 15*(1), 11-21.

Meiser, B. (2005). Psychological impact of genetic testing for cancer susceptibility: An update of the literature. *Psycho-Oncology, 14*(12), 1060-1074.

Metcalfe, A., Coad, J., Plumridge, G. M., Gill, P., & Farndon, P. (2008). Family communication between children and their parents about inherited genetic conditions: A meta-synthesis of the research. *European Journal of Human Genetics, 16*(10), 1193-1200.

Miller, S. M., McDaniel, S. H., Rolland, J. H., & Feetham, S. L. (Eds.). (2006). *Individuals, families, and the new era of genetics: Biopsychosocial perspectives.* New York: W. W. Norton & Company.

National Cancer Institute PDQ Genetics Editorial Board. (2011). *Risk assessment and counseling: Employment and insurance discrimination.* Retrieved from http://www.cancer.gov/cancertopics/pdq/genetics/risk-assessment-and-counseling/HealthProfessional/page6#Section_386

National Human Genome Research Institute. (2010). *The road to the $1,000 genome—A roundup of sequencing technology developments.* Retrieved from http://www.genome.gov/27540667

National Society of Genetic Counselors' Definition Task Force, Resta, R., Biesecker, B. B., Bennett, R. L., Blum, S., Hahn, S. E., Strecker, M. N., Williams, J. L. (2006). A new definition of genetic counseling: national society of genetic counselors' task force report. *Journal of Genetic Counseling, 15*(2), 77-83.

Office of Surveillance, Epidemiology, and Laboratory Services, Public Health Genomics, Centers for Disease Control and Prevention. (2010). *ACCE model list of 44 targeted questions aimed at a comprehensive review of genetic testing.* Retrieved from http://www.cdc.gov/genomics/gtesting/ACCE/acce_proj.htm

Olsen, S., Dudley-Brown, S., & McMullen, P. (2004). Case for blending pedigrees, genograms, and ecomaps: Nursing's contribution to the 'big picture'. *Nursing and Health Sciences, 6*(4), 295-308.

Pettersson, E., Lundeberg, J., & Ahmadian, A. (2009). Generations of sequencing technologies. *Genomics, 93*(2), 105-111.

Robson, M. E., Storm, C. D., Weitzel, J., Wollins, D. S., & Offit, K. (2010). American Society of Clinical Oncology policy statement update: Genetic and genomic testing for cancer susceptibility. *Journal of Clinical Oncology, 28*(5), 893-901.

Snyder, M., Jiang Du, J., & Gerstein, M. (2010). Personal genome sequencing: Current approaches and challenges. *Genes and Development, 24*, 423-431.

Stalker, H. J., Wilson, R., McCune, H., Gonzalez, J., Moffett, M., & Zori, R. T. (2006). Telegenetic medicine: Improved access to services in an underserved area. *Journal of Telemedicine and Telecare, 12*(4), 182-185.

Tercyak, K. P., Hensley Alford, S., Emmons, K. M., Lipkus, I. M., Wilfond, B. S., & McBride, C. M. (2011). Parents' attitudes toward pediatric genetic testing for common disease risk. *Pediatrics, 127*(5), e1288-1295.

Tischkowitz, M., & Rosser, E. (2004). Inherited cancer in children: Practical/ethical problems and challenges. *European Journal of Cancer, 40*, 2459-2470.

Wertz, D. C., Fanos, J. H., & Reilly, P. R. (1994). Genetic testing for children and adolescents. Who decides? *Journal of the American Medical Association, 272*(11), 875-881.

RESEARCH ADVOCACY IN CLINICAL NURSING

7

–Kim Mooney-Doyle, MSN, RN
Doctoral candidate, University of Pennsylvania School of Nursing

–Gwenyth R. Wallen, PhD, RN
Chief of Nursing Research and Translational Science,
National Institutes of Health Clinical Center

–Connie M. Ulrich, PhD, RN, FAAN
Associate Professor of Bioethics and Nursing
University of Pennsylvania School of Nursing
Secondary Appointment, Department of Medical Ethics and Health Policy
Senior Fellow, Leonard Davis Institute for Health Economics
New Courtland Center for Health and Transitions

Think About It!

- Clinical practice and clinical research are distinctly different aspects of patient care.

- Informed consent is an essential element of the ethical conduct of research and is an ongoing process.

- The ethical principles of respect for persons, beneficence, and justice can guide nurses in their daily care of patients enrolled in research.

Nurses often state that they go into nursing to make a significant difference in the lives of their patients and families. Actively diminishing the pain and suffering of those who are acutely, critically, or chronically ill is especially rewarding to them. Staff nurses on the front lines of health care delivery consistently assess and evaluate the physical and psychosocial needs of their patients. Research is not usually on the minds of practicing nurses, yet research is integral to improving patient-related outcomes. In fact, Willis and Grace (2011) argue that nurses are ethically responsible for understanding the science behind their patients' conditions, including learning about topics that advance the theoretical and empirical knowledge base of nursing practice. Additionally, Grady and Edgerly (2009) note that "in many settings, nurses are ethically responsible for contributing to both the promotion of good science and to the protection of the rights and welfare of patient subjects, a balance which requires knowledge, competence, advocacy, creativity, and close working relationships within the research and clinical teams" (p. 3).

Although nurse researchers are deeply involved in the research process and face considerable ethical challenges, this chapter is focused on staff nurses whose primary responsibility is at the bedside. At the bedside, individual clinical care of human subjects is often entangled with the procedures required by the research study. Balancing these two very different aspects of a patient's care—clinical care and clinical research—can create tension for bedside clinicians because of their primary advocacy obligations on behalf of the patient.

> ### Case Study 7.1
>
> A 50-year-old man (Mr. A) recently diagnosed with Parkinson's disease arrives on your unit, complaining of frequent hand tremors and an unstable gait that hinders him at work. During your conversation and exam, the patient asks your advice concerning an ongoing study on the genetic aspects of Parkinson's disease. The patient asks you if he would be a "good" candidate for the study and what benefit(s) he and his family might experience if he participated and a genetic component to the disease was discovered. In addition, he was also approached by another researcher who is investigating a drug that was initially approved for a different disease. Mr. A has also been told that the "new" drug might be helpful for patients with Parkinson's disease. He is worried about the possibility of receiving a placebo, and he isn't sure what it means for him if he does not receive the experimental drug. He is also concerned about how the study drug and his participation in the trial would improve his immediate problem of frequent tremors and unstable gait that impact his quality of life.

To have a discussion with Mr. A in the introductory case example, the nurse must be cognizant of several important facts:

- What is research, and how is it different from clinical practice?

- What are the basic elements of informed consent?

- Does Mr. A understand the research he is invited to participate in?

- What is the type of clinical research trial that Mr. A is considering (i.e., randomized placebo-controlled, observational, prevention, or screening trial)?

- What ethical codes of research conduct might be helpful in thinking through the research process?

- Are any special considerations associated with genetic research (i.e., concerns about privacy and confidentiality of data; whether individual genetic results will be provided to research participants, and whether family members will be recruited)?

- How does the nurse balance his or her advocacy role when patients are considering research participation and promote the patient's best interest?

Many clinical nurses work in institutions where research is central to the mission of that particular organization. For example, at the National Institutes of Health Clinical Center, the specialty of clinical research nursing is fundamental to the provision of care and includes five dimensions: clinical practice, study management, care coordination and continuity, human subjects protection, and contributing to the science. Each of these dimensions, however, is applicable to all bedside clinicians in most major health care institutions, because clinical nurses deliver the care that is needed to implement a clinical study or they might be in a position to coordinate and manage clinical trials on behalf of a principal investigator (Bevans, et al., 2011; Castro et al., 2011). In the case of Mr. A., the clinical nurse coordinating his care was simply asked to share her thoughts on research participation, but the response can have profound ethical implications, depending on the nurse's personal and professional concerns.

The Goals of Clinical Research and Clinical Care

Clinical research is an important societal mission that has the potential to advance the public's understanding of human health and illness. Historically, clinical research and clinical care have had a close relationship. Because both deal with the treatment of problems that are troublesome to individuals, families, and communities, inherent similarities will be present. For example, clinical research generally attempts to compare a new treatment to the standard of care treatment; therefore, the clinical care offered in a research trial should mirror or improve upon the usual standard of care offered in the clinical setting. Table 7.1 is a list of common terms and definitions used in clinical research that nurses should be familiar with.

Table 7.1   Table of Common Clinical Research Terms

Common Term	Definition
Principal Investigator (PI)	The principal investigator is the individual responsible for the overall scientific and ethical conduct of the research. This individual has both the authority and responsibility to direct the clinical trial, intellectually and logistically. This includes accountability for human subjects protection. In addition, the PI is responsible for making sure that the study is conducted in accordance with institutional, federal, state, and local laws and regulations.
Institutional Review Board (IRB)	1. A committee of physicians, statisticians, researchers, community advocates, and others that ensures that a clinical trial is ethical and that the rights of study participants are protected. All clinical trials in the United States must be approved by an IRB before they begin. 2. Every institution that conducts or supports biomedical or behavioral research involving human participants must, by federal regulation, have an IRB that initially approves and periodically reviews the research to protect the rights of human participants.
Adverse Event	An unwanted effect caused by the administration of drugs. Onset can be sudden or develop over time.
Clinical Trial	A clinical trial is a research study to answer specific questions about new therapies, vaccines, or new ways of using known treatments. Clinical trials (also called medical research and research studies) are used to determine whether new drugs or treatments are both safe and effective. Carefully conducted clinical trials are the fastest and safest way to find treatments that work in people. Trials are in four phases: Phase I tests a new drug or treatment in a small group; Phase II expands the study to a larger group of people; Phase III expands the study to an even larger group of people; and Phase IV takes place after the drug or treatment has been licensed and marketed.

Table 7.1 Table of Common Clinical Research Terms (cont.)

Common Term	Definition
Randomization	A method based on chance by which study participants are assigned to a treatment group. Randomization minimizes the differences among groups by equally distributing people with particular characteristics among all the trial arms. The researchers do not know which treatment is better. From what is known at the time, any one of the treatments chosen could be of benefit to the participant.
Placebo	A placebo is an inactive pill, liquid, or powder that has no treatment value. In clinical trials, experimental treatments are often compared with placebos to assess the treatment's effectiveness.
Equipoise	A state of genuine uncertainty on the part of the clinical investigators and expert medical community regarding the comparative therapeutic merits of each arm in a clinical trial (Freedman, 1987).

Sourced from Rozovsky & Adams, 2003

The goals of clinical research are distinctly different from clinical practice. The Belmont Report is a historical document that clarifies these distinctions and is important for understanding the ethical protections of human subjects in research (see Table 7.2; National Commission for the Protection of Human Subjects of Biomedical and Behavioral Research, 1979).

- The main goal of clinical research is to gain new knowledge with the hope of benefitting future individuals with the same affliction. It is a systematic process that uses a structured set of procedures to test specific hypotheses for the purpose of developing generalizable knowledge.

- Clinical care is provided with the goal of benefitting a particular person.

A difference also exists in how care is decided upon:

- In clinical research, the treatment offered to the patient-subject is often based upon the randomization process (a process where patient-subjects have an equal chance of receiving the experimental drug).

- In clinical care, the treatment offered is based upon a health care provider's judgment of a particular individual's needs.

In Mr. A's case, for example, assume that the purpose of the genetic-based research protocol is to better understand genetic susceptibility to Parkinson's disease. Importantly, the study has the potential to develop new targeted interventions for treatment of the disease in the future. Although Mr. A might derive immediate satisfaction in knowing that he potentially helped future patients diagnosed with Parkinson's disease, clinical research generally is not meant to directly benefit patient-subjects (although at times it does). Clinical research also offers the benefit of consistent, frequent monitoring by health care providers with expertise in the particular specialty. Still, participants in clinical research might not realize the benefits of the new intervention or therapy and might experience side effects from it as well. However, their participation can benefit future individuals afflicted with the same condition. On the other hand, clinical practice is expressly meant to benefit individual patients and includes those "interventions that are designed solely to enhance the well-being of an individual patient or client and that have a reasonable expectation of success" (National Commission for the Protection of Human Subjects of Biomedical and Behavioral Research, 1979). In other words, the focus of clinical research is on developing new knowledge, whereas the focus of clinical practice is on the care and treatment of an individual patient. The difference of focus means when a clinician performs research in a clinical setting, it can create some unique ethical dilemmas.

Table 7.2   Ethical Principles Outlined in the Belmont Report

ETHICAL PRINCIPLES	DEFINITIONS
Respect for Persons	Acknowledging a patient's right to autonomy in making decisions and choices about participating in research and protecting those with diminished autonomy.
Beneficence	An obligation to do no harm and to maximize the possible benefits and minimize the possible harms associated with research.
Justice	What is considered fair, due, or owed to persons; for example, genetic mutations or variations should not preclude individuals from equal access to employment or health care insurance.

Nurses often have a variety of roles in the conduct of research. At the bedside and in direct clinical care, they may be involved in recruiting participants, obtaining informed consent, answering participant questions, carrying out the study protocol, and collecting data (Christenberry & Miller, 2008). Nurse scientists and researchers, in addition to these responsibilities, design research protocols, implement human subjects' protections, analyze, and disseminate data from their research. Bedside nurses are expected to assess and evaluate the health care-related needs of their patients. As caregivers, though, they are also in a prime position to recognize any procedural irregularities, adverse events, or associated physical, emotional, and psychosocial aspects of their patient-subject's research participation (Grady & Edgerly, 2009). In their study on competing commitments in clinical trials, Lidz and colleagues (2009) reported that clinicians (including nurses) often feel tension between clinical research and clinical practice care procedures when advocating for patient-subjects. In fact, more than half (52%) of their respondents indicated a situation whereby the study protocol prohibited the use of a medication that was deemed beneficial by clinicians to the patient-subject. Consequently, 28% of these respondents reported that at least on one occasion, the restricted medication was given to the patient-subject. Although clinicians might feel as though they are acting in the best interest of their patients, deviating from a research protocol can have serious consequences for the overall integrity of the research and the conclusions that are drawn. For example, in a study testing the efficacy of an integrative approach to symptom management in the ICU, the bedside nurse noticed that her patient was in pain. Because of this, she chose not to approach the eligible patient to participate in the clinical trial, because she felt as though the research would be an additional burden and she felt obligated to diminish the patient's pain and suffering. By doing so, the nurse might have compromised the study and, importantly, denied the participant an autonomous choice—an essential component of what makes research ethical.

Informed Consent and the History of Human Subjects Protection

Informed consent is a historical, ethical, and legal document for the protection of human subjects and a necessary component of ethical research. Throughout the 20th century, different events in America and around the world signaled the need for guidance in research with human participants. Although Figure 7.1 starts in the early 20th century, some form of obtaining informed consent can be considered an ancient practice because of physician obligations expressed in the Hippocratic Oath. The notion of written informed consent dates back to 1900, when then-Army physician Walter Reed obtained consent from patients with yellow fever (Jefford & Moore, 2008). The following section is a more detailed description of the various events that mark the evolution of research ethics with humans in the 20th century. In addition, the historical cases continue to provide relevance and guidance for everyday nursing practice in the following ways:

- Informed consent represents the autonomous choice of an individual and is an essential element of ethical research.

- Every patient-subject has the right to withdraw from research without penalty. In other words, treatment cannot be denied for patient-subject withdrawal or refusal to participate.

- Research must be voluntary and free from undue influence.

- Regardless of gender, age, race/ethnicity or other characteristics, all eligible patients have the right to participate equally.

- Certain populations are deemed "vulnerable" in research (i.e., pregnant women, children, prisoners) and require further safeguards (National Institutes of Heath, 2005).

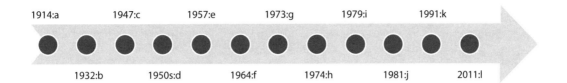

a. Justice Cardoza (USA) laid out basic principles for laws regulating informed consent in USA and other nations.

b. Start of the Tuskegee Syphilis Study.

c. Nuremberg Code initiated after the Nuremberg trial of those responsible for Nazi medical experimentation.

d. Thalidomide tragedy.

e. California law created around an informed consent standard for clinical care.

f. Declaration of Helsinki.

g. End of Tuskegee Syphilis Study.

h. Passage of National Research Act in response to atrocities of Tuskegee.

i. Belmont Report issued as a direct result of the National Research Act.

j. DHHS & FDA issued code of federal regulations (CFR).

k. Common Rule adopted.

l. Common Rule updated.

Figure 7.1 History of current clinical and research ethics and resulting codes and guidelines.

Schloendorff v. Society of New York Hospital

In 1914, Justice Cardoza identified the basic principle that shaped American and international law regarding research ethics in the case *Schloendorff v. Society of New York Hospital,* issued by the New York Court of Appeals. "Every human being of adult years and sound mind has a right to determine what should be done with his [or her] own body," he stated (Jefford & Moore, 2008). Each individual has a right to determine what is in his or her best interest (ethical principle of autonomy or respect for persons).

From 1932-1973, the "Tuskegee Study of Untreated Syphilis in Black Men" (U.S. Public Health Service in collaboration with the Tuskegee Institute), investigated the natural progression of syphilis in 600 African-American men (400 with syphilis and 200 without it). The study violated basic ethical principles of informed consent and respect for persons, as the men were never informed of the true nature and purpose of the study, provided with penicillin to treat the disease when it became available, or told that they could withdraw from the study at any point (http://www.cdc.gov/tuskegee/timeline.htm).

In 1947, the Nuremberg Code specifically addressed the need for research participation to be voluntary and for the greater public good. This code was a direct result of the Nazi medical experiments during World War II (http://ohsr.nih.gov/guidelines).

In the 1950s, Thalidomide was a sedative prescribed to control nausea and aid in sleep control during pregnancy. The drug was not approved in the United States and ultimately was linked to numerous birth defects and infant deaths. This event led the way for the Kefauver Amendments to the Food, Drug, and Cosmetic Act in 1962 to ensure greater oversight and safety of drugs marketed to the public.

In 1964, the Declaration of Helsinki was commissioned by the World Medical Association (WMA) to provide guidance to physicians in the ethical conduct of research. It provided the first discussions surrounding the role of physicians as investigators and the intersection of clinical care and clinical research (http://ohsr.nih.gov/guidelines).

In 1974, The National Research Act was promulgated following the Tuskegee Syphilis Study. This act authorized the creation of the National Commission for the Protection of Human Subjects of Biomedical and Behavioral Research (Emanuel & Menikoff, 2011). And, the Belmont Report was born from the meetings of this National Commission. This report identified three basic ethical principles that should underlie all research with human subjects and their application throughout the research process: respect for persons, beneficence, and justice (http://ohsr.nih.gov/ guidelines [See Table 7.1 earlier in the chapter]).

In 1981, The Department of Health and Human Services (DHHS) of the United States adopted the recommendations of the Belmont Report to expand its regulatory protections. This became known as the Code of Federal Regulation, Title 45, Part 46 (which is better known as 45 CFR 46; Emanuel & Menikoff, 2011). 45 CFR 46 has wide-reaching implications for research within the United States and abroad because of its influence on federally funded clinical research or research conducted by U.S. investigators. This code contains several subparts that delineate limits to risks of research participation that might be incurred by certain populations deemed *vulnerable*. This includes children; prisoners; and pregnant women, their fetuses, and their infants; as well as adults who cannot provide consent. See the National Institutes of Health, Subpart B, C, and D for further information.

In 1991, Subpart A of the Code of Federal Regulations, Title 45, Part 46, identified requirements for informed consent in research and the conduct of institutional review boards. This was adopted across 14 government agencies and is better known as "the Common Rule" (Emanuel & Menikoff, 2011).

In 2011, updates to the Common Rule have been proposed to streamline the regulatory process to link the highest levels of scrutiny with the studies that pose the greatest risk to participants, to protect privacy and confidentiality, and to reform the informed consent process for understandability (http://www.hhs.gov/ohrp/humansubjects/anprmchangetable.pdf.pdf).

Case Study 7.2

Mr. W is a 90-year-old metastatic melanoma patient. He lives alone but is currently hospitalized for severe headaches and dehydration because of nausea and vomiting. He has been asked to participate in a clinical trial testing a new neuroimaging technique. You were present when the clinical investigator obtained a signed informed consent from him when he was first admitted. However, when you visit Mr. W today and ask him if he is ready to begin the study tomorrow, he looks at you blankly and seems to have no idea what you are talking about.

Informed Consent

Rather than a single, discrete event, informed consent is an ongoing process between the researcher and the participant and requires people to decide freely about their choices and understand the elements of the research they are undertaking, and it protects their right to self-determination (Flory, Wendler, & Emanuel, 2008).

In the preceding scenario, the nurse is morally obligated to assess Mr. W's decision-making capacity, because he appears to not understand that he will be participating in research. Informed consent involves three main components: voluntariness, disclosure of information, and assessment of a subject's capacity (understanding being one part of capacity). A person's abilities to make a decision, or decisional capacity, is measured by assessing his or her capacities to understand, appreciate, reason, and express a choice (Grisso & Appelbaum, 1998). In the preceding case, the nurse could assess Mr. W's understanding of the trial by asking the following questions:

- How well does Mr. W understand the research trial in which he has enrolled?

- What does Mr. W understand the research question under investigation to be?

- Can Mr. W express what the investigators are planning to do in the trial?

- Can Mr. W express other critical aspects of the trial?

Improving informed consent procedures in prospective patient-subjects is of critical importance for all significant parties involved in the research process. Extensive research has shown that patient-subject characteristics such as poor education, limited literacy, and cognitive impairment can impact a patient-subject's decision-making (Agre et al., 2003; Agre & Rapkin, 2003; Cassileth, Lusk, Miller, & Hurwitz, 1982; Joffe, Cook, Cleary, Clark, & Weeks, 2000; Sachs et al., 2003; Siminoff, 2003). Many studies have also reported gaps in subjects' knowledge and recall of information associated with research enrollment (Agre et al., 2003; Agre & Rapkin, 2003; Siminoff, 2003; Sachs et al., 2003). In addition, although informed consent is an essential element in ethical research, it is not sufficient (Emanuel, Wendler, Grady, 2000). Barriers to informed consent include the language, format, and length of the consent document; the severity of illness or clinical care needs of the patient; and other aspects of the hospital environment that impact the patient's cognitive abilities. Unfortunately, informed consent documents are often long, hard to understand, and at a greater than high school readability level. Most documents should be at a fourth- to sixth-grade reading level (Paasche-Orlow, Taylor, & Brancati, 2003). Nurses must continually assess that their patients have an adequate decision-making ability to provide informed consent and recognize that hospitalization or other inpatient procedures might alter their decision-making abilities.

Who Is Vulnerable in Research and Why?

Certain populations are afforded increased protection in research because of the potential risks to their participation, their position in society, the potential threat to their civil liberties, and, ultimately, their inability to fully consent and understand the implications of their research participation. As previously discussed in this chapter, vulnerable populations as described in the Code of Federal Regulations include pregnant women, their fetuses and their neonates; prisoners; and children and adults who cannot provide informed consent.

Case Study 7.3

Abigail is a 12-year-old patient with osteogenesis imperfecta, a genetic bone disorder causing extremely fragile bones. She gets enrolled in a clinical trial that will involve multiple blood draws, x-rays, and bone scans during a week-long hospital stay. Though the study team thinks that Abigail seems to understand the rationale behind joining the study, Abigail is very distant and apprehensive when she comes in for study visits. The clinical nurse overhears Abigail crying to her parents over all the diagnostic procedures, including the blood draws, and then hears the parents tell Abigail all the things that they will buy her if she completes the study. The nurse is worried that Abigail's participation is not voluntary, and she is being forced to participate by her parents.

Abigail represents one of the populations afforded additional protections because she is a child. In this case, the nurse is placed in a difficult ethical situation as she overhears Abigail's distress. Some of the ethical concerns might include: Would it be professional—and ethical—to talk to Abigail's parents about what she overheard? Should she say anything to the individuals conducting the study? What does the nurse say to Abigail, if anything? Finally, the nurse might wonder if a 12-year-old is able to reasonably decide whether she wants to continue in the research study and at what age can children provide assent to research.

There are several options for the nurse in this case. First, she is professionally and morally obligated to follow through on what she heard, but she might do this in several different ways, depending on her comfort level and relationship with the child and parents. We list a few suggestions below:

- Directly speak with Abigail to better understand her concerns about research participation and any pressures she might be experiencing. The perspectives and input of children should be included in concert with their parents'. In this situation, the parents might be reacting out of fear for their child's health and well-being.

- Organize a unit-level meeting of all primary members of Abigail's research and clinical care team to delineate the ethical issues, allowing all voices to be represented and heard.

- Contact the ethics committee to provide a formal consultation regarding the situation. An ethics consultant can foster a discussion of the ethical issue(s) with the patient and parents, as well as the clinicians and research team.

- Contact the pediatric psychologist or psychiatrist on staff to speak with Abigail and her parents about Abigail's distress.

"Because children are vulnerable, and especially because research might not provide a direct benefit to them, the issue of consent to their participation becomes paramount" (Cassidy & Fleischman, 1996, p. 189). Children have not reached the legal age for consent and, therefore, parents are responsible for acting in the best interest of their child. Today, children generally ages 7 and older, depending on level of maturity, state regulations, and institutional review board considerations, can participate in research. They provide what is called *pediatric assent* along with *parental permission*. In *pediatric assent*, all elements of the informed consent document are written at a developmentally appropriate level for children (see the following sidebar).

> ### Risk Levels and Pediatric Research
>
> Federal guidelines for the protection of children enrolled in research are included under 45 CFR 46 Subpart D. Risk in studies that involve children is evaluated by classifying the research as follows: 1) research not involving greater than minimal risk; 2) research involving greater than minimal risk but presenting the prospect of direct benefit to the individual subjects (National Institutes of Health, 2005); 3) research involving greater than minimal risk and no prospect of direct benefit to individual subjects, but likely to yield generalizable knowledge about the subject's disorder or condition (National Institutes of Health, 2005); or 4) research not otherwise approvable, which presents an opportunity to understand, prevent, or alleviate a serious problem affecting the health or welfare of children (National Institutes of Health, 2005). http://ohsr.od.nih.gov/guidelines/45cfr46.html

Research Ethics and Advocacy in Clinical Practice

In the previous sections, we discuss some of the challenges of research participation, specifically focusing on issues surrounding informed consent, the misuse of human participants, and the public's fear and mistrust of the research enterprise. But, what makes research ethical? In their sentinel work, Emanuel, Wendler, and Grady (2000) outline seven critical elements of ethical research. This includes the importance of the research question under study, rigorous methods to answer the question(s), fair subject selection, minimizing the risks and maximizing the benefits, independent review and informed consent, and finally, respect for potential and enrolled subjects (i.e., privacy and confidentiality of information, the right to withdraw at any time, and informing subjects of new information that might arise during their research participation). To assist their patients and to better understand the research process, clinical research nurses can ask a variety of questions to clarify their particular concerns. We list a few of these below:

- What is the research question? Is it addressing a significant health-related problem? Why is my patient eligible?

- What are the scientific goals of the study?

- What are the risks and benefits of the study?

- What are the specific procedural aspects of the protocol? In other words, what is the research team asking the patient to do?

- Has the study been approved by the appropriate institutional review board or any other research committee that is required?

- Who is conducting the research?

- Is there a need for additional safeguards because of the vulnerability of the population? (i.e., surrogate consent, pediatric assent)

- What if the patient experiences an adverse event? As the bedside nurse, what is my role if this happens?

Research can benefit subjects in both tangible and intangible ways. In fact, many study participants hope for some personal benefit to their participation. Several authors seek to reframe the way we view research participation and participants' ability to exert their agency and self-determination. For example, Schaefer, Emanuel, and Wertheimer (2009) consider that individuals have an obligation to participate in clinical research in order to contribute to the "public good of generalizable medical knowledge," and this view is based in the ethical principle of beneficence. The authors posit that because clinical research produces knowledge, which is advantageous to all members of society, each person has an obligation to support the system through participation (Schaefer, et al., 2009). Nurse clinicians are in key positions to support research because they are not only direct caregivers for patients who are often enrolled in research protocols, but also are responsible for assessing, implementing, and evaluating research-related procedures. This means, however, that nurses must understand the differences between clinical care and clinical research, be prepared to address research-related questions that might arise, and discuss any ethical concerns.

Conclusion

Is there a way to balance patient advocacy in clinical care, while at the same time protecting patient-subjects enrolled in clinical research? Ulrich, Wallen, and Grady (2002) ask this compelling question to help nurses think about who is vulnerable in research and to remember that the goals of the patients and families we serve should direct the care they provide to them. Therefore, it is not the nurse's decision whether or not patients participate in clinical research. Nurses can assist patient-subjects, however, by making sure that the environment is as accommodating as possible, so that patient-subjects have the opportunity to discuss the research process and ask any questions that they might have. In addition, nurses must remember that not all individuals are vulnerable in the same way. Many ill or distressed patients have adequate capacity to choose or decline participation in clinical research; supporting this ability is akin to supporting patient autonomy and self-determination (Ulrich et al., 2002). Though some groups of individuals are indeed more vulnerable than others, this does not preclude their participation in clinical research. This might also require that nurses caring for critically ill research patient-subjects remain particularly vigilant and thoughtful as they provide clinical care, while maintaining the integrity of the clinical trial and supporting an ongoing informed consent process.

Ethical advocacy, both in clinical research and clinical care, requires that nurses in all settings "safeguard vulnerable groups from potential exploitation and risky research; maximize their capacity for self-determination; and protect their welfare" (Ulrich et al., 2002, p. 72). Ethical practice in either realm is heavily dependent upon the integrity of investigators, other individuals involved in the research process, and clinicians providing direct clinical care.

Talk About It!

- How does research impact your clinical practice? What are the challenges you face in implementing research at the bedside?

- In thinking about the case study with 12 year old Abigail, consider the perspective/position of her parents. Why might they try to influence her decision with gifts? What would you do if you were Abigail's mom or dad? What would you want the adults in your life to do if you were Abigail?

- Thinking about informed consent, how have you supported your patients enrolled in research? Have you ever intervened to assist patients in understanding the research protocol? If so, in what way(s)?

References

Agre, P., Campbell, F. A., Goldman, B. D., Boccia, M. L., Kass, N., McCullough, L. B., ... Wirshing. D. (2003). Improving informed consent: The medium is not the message. *IRB: Ethics and Human Research, 25*(5), S11-S19.

Agre, P., & Rapkin, B. (2003). Improving informed consent: A comparison of four consent tools. *IRB: Ethics and Human Research, 25*(6), 1-7.

Bevans, M., Hastings, C., Wehrlen, L., Cusack, G., Matlock, A. M., Miller-Davis, C., ...Wallen, G.R. (2011). Defining clinical research nursing practice: Results of a role delineation study. *Clinical and Translational Science. 4*(6), 421-427.

Cassidy, R.C., & Fleischman, A.R. (1996). *Pediatric ethics-From principles to practice.* Amsterdam: The Netherlands: Harwood Academic Publishers.

Cassileth, B. R., Lusk, E. J., Miller, D. S., & Hurwitz, S. (1982). Attitudes toward clinical trials among patients and the public. *Journal of the American Medical Association, 248*(8), 968-970.

Castro, K., Bevans, M., Miller-Davis, C., Cusack, G., Loscalzo, F., Matlock, A. M., ... Hastings, C. (2011). Validating the clinical research nursing domain of practice. *Oncology Nursing Forum, 38*(2), E72-80.

Centers for Disease Control and Prevention. (2011). *U.S. Public Health Service syphilis study at Tuskegee.: The Tuskegee Timeline.* Retrieved from http://www.cdc.gov/tuskegee/timeline.htm

Christenberry, T. L., & Miller, M. R. (2008). A strategy for learning principles and elements of informed consent. *Nurse Educator, 33*(2), 75-78.

Department of Health and Human Services. (2005). *Research involving children: HHS regulatory requirements for research involving children described in subpart D.* Retrieved from http://grants.nih.gov/grants/policy/hs/children.htm

Department of Health and Human Services. (2011). *Advanced notice of proposed rule making for revisions to the common rule.* Retrieved from http://www.hhs.gov/ohrp/humansubjects/anprmchangetable.pdf.pdf

Emanuel, E., Wendler, D., & Grady, C. (2000). What makes clinical research ethical? *Journal of the American Medical Association, 283*(20), 2701-2711.

Emanuel, E. J., & Menikoff, J. (2011). Reforming the regulations governing research with human subjects. *New England Journal of Medicine, 365*(12), 1145-1151.

Flory, J., Wendler, D., & Emanuel, E. (2008). Empirical issues in informed consent research. In E. Emanuel, C. Grady, R. Crouch, R. Lie, F. Miller, & D. Wendler (Eds.), *The Oxford textbook of clinical research ethic.* (pp. 645–660). New York: Oxford University Press.

Freedman, B. (1987). Equipoise and the ethics of clinical research. *New England Journal of Medicine, 317*(3), 141-145.

Grady, C., & Edgerly, M. (2009). Science, technology, and innovation: Nursing responsibilities in clinical research. *Nursing Clinics of North America, 44*(4), 471-481.

Grisso, T., & Appelbaum, P. S. (1998). *Thinking about competence. Assessing competence to consent to treatment. A guide for physicians and other health professionals.* New York: Oxford University Press.

Jefford, M., & Moore, R. (2008). Improvement of informed consent and the quality of consent documents. *Lancet Oncology, 9*(5),485-493.

Joffe, S., Cook, E. F., Cleary, P. D., Clark, J. W., & Weeks, J. C. (2000). Quality of informed consent in cancer cliinical trials: A cross-sectional survey. *Lancet, 358*(9295): 1772-1777.

Lidz, C.W., Appelbaum, P. S., Joffe, S., Albert K., Rosenbaum, J., & Simon, L. (2009). Competing commitments in clinical trials. *IRB: Ethics and Human Research, 31*(5), 1-6.

National Commission for the Protection of Human Subjects of Biomedical and Behavioral Research. (1979). *The Belmont Report.* Washington, DC: U.S. Government Printing Office.

National Institutes of Health. (2005). *Regulations and ethical guidelines: Title 45 code of Federal regulations, Part 46 Protection of Human Subjects.* Retrieved from http://ohsr.od.nih.gov/guidelines/45cfr46.html

National Institutes of Health. (2008). *Glossary of clinical trials terms.* Retrieved from http://clinicaltrials.gov/ct2/info/glossary

Paasche-Orlow, M. K., Taylor, H. A., & Brancati, F. L. (2003). Readability standards for informed-consent: Forms as compared with actual readability. *New England Journal of Medicine, 348*(8), 721-726.

Rozovsky, F. A., & Adams, R. K. (2003). Clinical trials and human research: A practical guide to regulatory compliance. San Francisco, CA: John Wiley & Sons.

Sachs, G. A., Hougham, G. W., Sugarman, J., Agre, P., Broome, M., Geller, G., … Weiss, A. (2003). Conducting empirical research on informed consent. *IRB: Ethics & Human Research, 25*(5), S4-S10.

Schaefer, G. O., Emanuel, E. J., & Wertheimer, A. (2009). The obligation to participate in biomedical research. *Journal of the American Medical Association, 302*(1), 67-72.

Siminoff, L. A. (2003). Toward improving the informed consent process in research with humans. *IRB: Ethics and Human Research. 25*(5), S1-S3.

Ulrich, C., Wallen, G., & Grady, C. (2002). Guest editorial: Research vulnerability and patient advocacy: Balance seeking perspectives for the clinical nurse scientist? *Nursing Research, 51*(2), 71.

Willis, D. G., & Grace, P. J. (2011). The applied philosopher-scientist: Intersections among phenomenological research, nursing science, and theory as a basis for practice aimed at facilitating boys' healing from being bullied. *Advances in Nursing Science, 34*(1), 19-28.

ETHICS IN SPECIALIZED NURSING CARE

II

ETHICAL ISSUES IN CRITICAL CARE 8

–Mindy B. Zeitzer, PhD, MBE, RN
Adjunct Professor
Thomas Jefferson University, School of Nursing

Think About It!

- Recognizing the ethical issue you are experiencing is important. If you are feeling conflicted over a patient care issue that is related to a value, moral, or ethic, you are experiencing an ethical issue.

- Consider how to approach ethical issues and what avenues are available to you within your unit and within your hospital. Familiarizing yourself with these before experiencing ethical issues is beneficial.

- Decide how you are going to deal with the issue and act on it.

- Remember to assess and reflect on how the issue was dealt with and how you ultimately feel about the situation.

Critical-care nursing includes caring for critically and acutely ill patients who can range from neonates to geriatrics in a general or specific critical-care unit (CCU) or emergency department. Critical-care nurses care for a broad range of patients suffering from various diseases or injury-related illnesses. Needless to say, critical care is complex; it typically includes many types of technology, raising an increasing number of ethical questions. In addition, critical-care nurses care for the sickest patients, many of whom are at the end of their lives. This creates a stressful atmosphere for families, who must often watch their loved one undergo intense hospitalization while often needing to make immediate and difficult decisions related to the loved one's care. Nurses working in critical-care units often deal with a multitude of ethical issues related to these factors. Being able to recognize ethical issues, formulate a plan, take action, and cope emotionally are important tasks for all critical-care nurses to absorb. This information is vital to their personal and professional well-being. This chapter discusses some typical ethical issues critical-care nurses encounter, their effects, and steps on how to tackle ethical problems.

> ### Case Study 8.1
>
> Lisa has been a critical-care nurse in the surgical trauma intensive care unit for 5 years. Currently, she is caring for a patient who has been on the unit for 1 month. Her patient, Rochelle, is a 73-year-old who has diabetes and was an unrestrained passenger in a motor vehicle collision. She suffered a massive brain bleed, a fractured pelvis, multiple contusions, and a hemopneumothorax. She has undergone multiple surgeries and is septic. Her condition continues to deteriorate, and the likelihood of full or partial recovery is slim. The health care team questions her ability to maintain a meaningful life. Rochelle has a 78-year-old husband and three grown children with families of their own. Her husband relates that she has expressed in the past that she would "not want to live like this," though she has no written advance directives. Rochelle's husband and her children insist that everything possible be done, at all costs. They are not willing to "let her go and give up." Her nurse, Lisa, is concerned that her patient is suffering and that her verbally expressed wishes are not being followed.

Situations such as Case Study 8.1 occur frequently in critical-care units. Lisa must balance her professional obligations of advocating for her patient and trying to follow her expressed wishes while also respecting the family's decisions for care. At the same time, she must adhere to her own personal values. Lisa is encountering many ethical issues in this scenario, including concerns about the absence of an advance directive, her patient's right to autonomy, and whether she is adding to the suffering of her patient by prolonging the patient's life when care seems futile. How can Lisa most effectively deal with this situation? What resources are available to her to help her through these issues? These are questions critical-care nurses encounter frequently and should be able to answer confidently when confronting ethical issues such as in the above case study.

Ethical Issues Critical-Care Nurses Encounter

The ethical issues nurses encounter in the critical-care setting are broad-based because they occur in a variety of patient settings (i.e., emergency department, operating room, intensive care unit) and within a myriad of complex relationships. These issues might arise within the nurse-physician relationship, the patient-family relationship, or even between the family and the health care team (Zeitzer, 2010). Whenever those involved have disagreements on goals of care, conflicts can occur. For example, suppose the family wants to continue care when the patient has expressed the wish to discontinue aggressive treatments (Hough, 2008; Zeitzer, 2010). Or conversely, what if the family wants to continue aggressive therapies, but the health care team deems it futile and ethically unacceptable? Problems could also be related to a particular department, the hospital where the nurse is employed, or even the health care system as a whole. For example, the resources needed to provide quality care might not be available because of cost containment pressures or inadequate staffing (Hough, 2008; Zeitzer, 2010). No matter where the issue arises or who is involved, the nurse is likely to feel caught between advocating for her patients' best interest and following hospital rules and regulations or other professional and personal mandates.

Critical care is unique because new and ever-changing technologies are frequently integrated into patient care. This situation often generates ethical issues that involve balancing the cost versus the benefit of the treatment while considering the patient's overall recovery and quality of life. Unique issues arising at the end of life include surrogate decision-making, evaluation of the futility of treatment, and the allocation of expensive, scarce resources. Informed consent, quality of life, and Do Not Resuscitate (DNR) orders often come into play as well, causing conflict within the care setting. Table 8.1 provides a list of common categories of ethical issues, with some examples of problems nurses frequently encounter in critical care.

Table 8.1   Common Ethical Issues Encountered by Critical-Care Nurses

Category of Ethical Issues	Examples of Specific Issues
Issues involving patients and families	Life-prolonging aggressive therapies and their good or harm to the patient Pain control: *Over/under medicating *Medicating terminally ill with possibility of hastening death Patient's right to autonomy Continuing aggressive treatments in futile situations DNR orders Withholding/withdrawing life support Overexposing patient to radiation Lack of informed consent Not telling the truth to patients or families/giving false hope Enrolling patients in research Organ donation *Starting treatment to make organs more viable *Presuming consent
Issues involving other staff	Questionable or inappropriate orders Not respecting patient's autonomy or wishes Gender or power issues Differing goals/opinions Nurses being disrespected Professional accountability
Issues involving resource allocation	Providing futile care and continuing the use of resources Inadequate staffing Ability to provide quality with cost containment Managed care
Issues involving communication problems	With patients With families With other nurses With physicians With administration

Sourced from Alt-White & Pranulis, 2006; Hough, 2008; Meltzer & Huckabay, 2004; Redman & Fry, 2000; Richmond & Ulrich, 2007; Zeitzer, 2010.
List not conclusive

Most ethical problems tend to be categorized among the existing bioethical principles: autonomy, beneficence, nonmaleficence, and justice (Beauchamp & Childress, 2001). These four principles are norms that serve as guidelines for professional ethics. Autonomy can be explained as the right to self-determination. Beneficence takes into consideration how the nurse "does good" for her patient, whereas nonmaleficence obligates the nurse to do no harm. Justice is an ethical principle that guides the fair distribution of benefit, risk, and cost. Zeitzer (2010) found that most ethical issues encountered in the emergency department during the resuscitation of the injured patient involved some element of these four categories. Though categorizing particular ethical issues does not always directly benefit the nurse dealing with them, learning to identify them and knowing how to deal with them are of benefit.

PURPOSE EXERCISE: CONSIDER AND WRITE YOUR ANSWERS TO THE FOLLOWING QUESTIONS

Think of ethical issues that you frequently encounter on your unit.

1. How are these issues currently handled?

2. Have you been satisfied with how they are handled in the past?

3. Think about what you can do differently to improve the manner in which ethical issues are dealt.

Effects of Ethical Issues in Critical Care

When encountering an ethical issue, nurses must resist the temptation to ignore it and must instead confront it in a professional manner. Such confrontation is important for nurses' health and well-being, as well as for the improvement of the system. Ethical issues can ultimately lead to moral distress, which has various negative effects on nurses. Moral distress occurs when a person knows the action he or she ought to take, but is prevented from doing so. For nurses, institutional constraints often prohibit the right course of action (Jameton, 1984).

Moral distress can have multiple negative effects, including the nurse experiencing burnout and leaving her current position, her specialty, or even the nursing profession. Furthermore, moral distress can cause feelings of anger, frustration, and guilt (Wilkinson, 1988). The American Association of Critical-Care Nurses (AACN; 2004) recognizes moral distress as a critical problem for nurses and one that needs immediate attention. When unaddressed, moral distress "restricts nurses' ability to provide optimal patient care and to find job satisfaction" (AACN, 2004, p. 1). The AACN suggests a model of the "4A's" to address moral distress. The 4A's of ask, affirm, assess, and act help instruct nurses on how to overcome the moral distress they experience. See Figure 8.1 for Model of the 4A's.

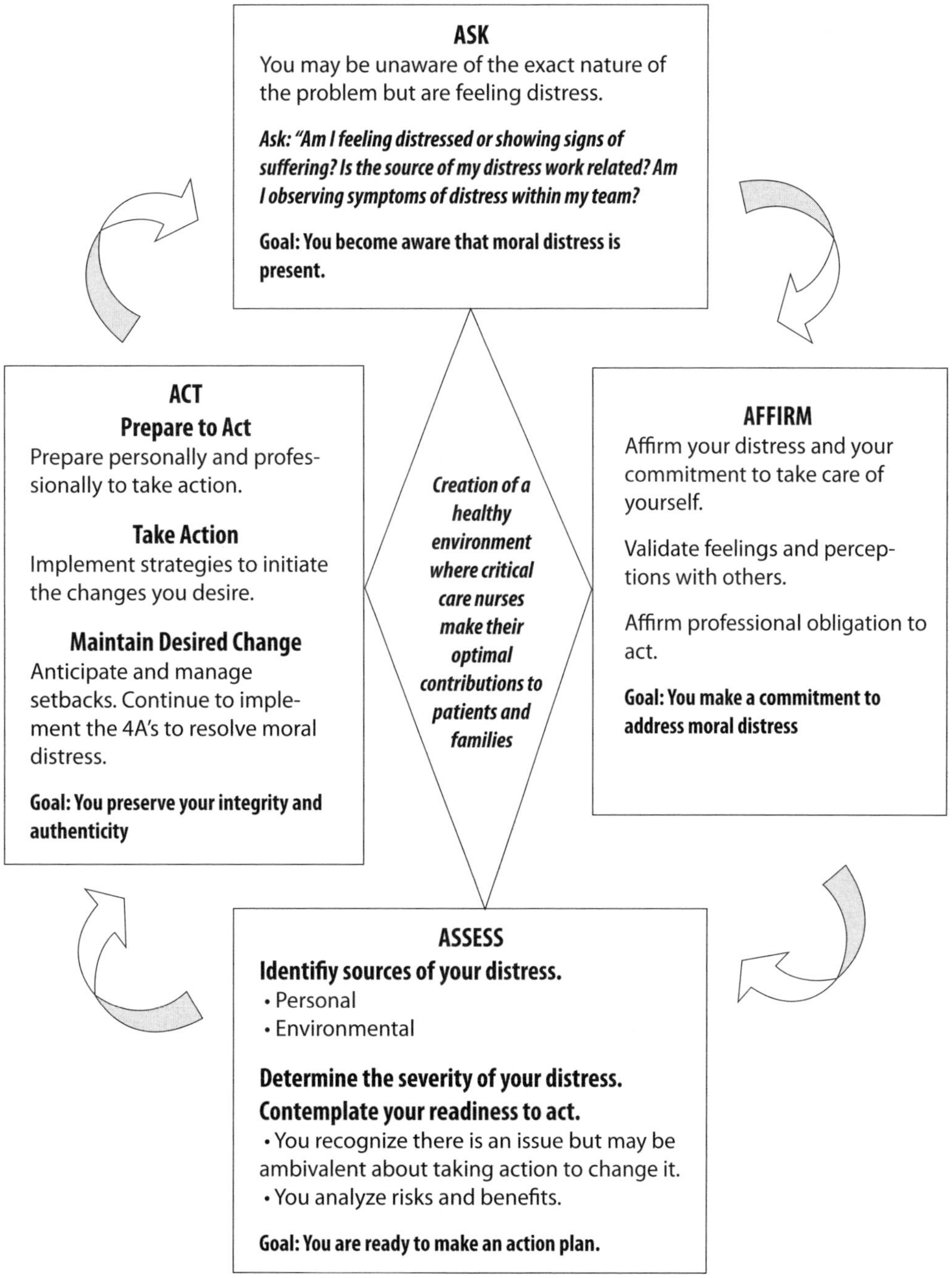

ASK

You may be unaware of the exact nature of the problem but are feeling distress.

Ask: "Am I feeling distressed or showing signs of suffering? Is the source of my distress work related? Am I observing symptoms of distress within my team?

Goal: You become aware that moral distress is present.

ACT
Prepare to Act
Prepare personally and professionally to take action.

Take Action
Implement strategies to initiate the changes you desire.

Maintain Desired Change
Anticipate and manage setbacks. Continue to implement the 4A's to resolve moral distress.

Goal: You preserve your integrity and authenticity

Creation of a healthy environment where critical care nurses make their optimal contributions to patients and families

AFFIRM

Affirm your distress and your commitment to take care of yourself.

Validate feelings and perceptions with others.

Affirm professional obligation to act.

Goal: You make a commitment to address moral distress

ASSESS
Identifiy sources of your distress.
• Personal
• Environmental

Determine the severity of your distress.
Contemplate your readiness to act.
• You recognize there is an issue but may be ambivalent about taking action to change it.
• You analyze risks and benefits.

Goal: You are ready to make an action plan.

Figure 8.1 Model of AACN's 4As to rise above moral distress
Reprinted with permission from AACN; Rushton & Westphal, 2004.

Some nurses explained that to cope with their moral distress, they left their units to find better working conditions, they worked fewer hours, they left nursing, or they blamed administration and the hospital system and avoided patient interaction (Kelly, 1998). All of these are devastating consequences that greatly affect patient care, the nursing profession, and the health care system. Moral distress has been shown to have many causes:

- The feeling that the patients are being treated as objects to meet institutional requirements (Holly, 1993)

- Observations of patients' pain and suffering (Raines, 2000)

- Withdrawal of treatment without nurse participation in the decision (Fry, Harvey, Hurley, & Foley, 2002)

- Poor pain management

- Disregard for patients' choices about accepting or refusing treatment

- The failure to fully inform patients and their families about treatment options (Viney, 1996)

Many of these situations involve nurses' inability to change care given to patients because of physicians or other health care providers dictating treatment goals, often leaving the nurses feeling powerless (Holly, 1993; Viney, 1996).

In addition to moral distress, ethical issues have been shown to have a plethora of other effects on nurses. Emotionally, the nurses feel angry, disappointed, ashamed, frustrated, or powerless, and some-times begin avoiding their emotions altogether (Zeitzer, 2010). Physically, nurses develop stress and even headaches (2010). Nurses relate that their lives, as well as their professional roles, are affected by the ethi-cal problems they experience in the workplace.

All of the effects of ethical issues discussed are devastating and ultimately lead to poor patient care, poor personal well-being of nurses, and fewer nurses in the workforce. Because of this, ethical issues need to be addressed in a timely manner by a person who is directly involved: the nurse.

 PURPOSE EXERCISE: CONSIDER AND WRITE YOUR ANSWERS TO THE FOLLOWING QUESTIONS

1. Have you ever felt moral distress?

2. How did it affect your life and/or work practices?

Dealing With Ethical Issues

Encountering an ethical issue is difficult for nurses both professionally and personally; thus, knowing how to deal with the issue is imperative. Primarily, nurses need to be able to recognize the issue and know whether the problem is ethical in nature. Additionally, nurses need to know appropriate steps to take in dealing with the issue and need to be aware of the avenues available to help resolve the problem. The following sections address these essential topics.

Recognizing Ethical Issues

When confronted with an ethical issue, nurses typically feel conflicted. Ulrich, Hamric, and Grady (2010) explain that ethical issues can arise in any situation where profound questions of what is morally right or wrong exist. For nurses, this can occur when they are involved in situations that cause some sort of suffering or personal conflict, leading to reactions of anxiety, guilt, doubt, or anger. Some questions nurses can ask to determine whether the problem is an ethical issue might include:

1. Do you feel conflicted? Does the conflict involve a disagreement between important values? Perhaps between a personal value and a treatment goal? Do you feel a moral objection to what has taken/is taking/will be taking place?

2. Is the problem ethical in nature? Are you using words such as *ought, should, right, wrong, good,* or *bad* when you describe the situation or how you are feeling (Jameton, 1984)? Does the problem fit within one of the four ethical principles: autonomy, beneficence, nonmaleficence, or justice? (Though determining whether the issue fits within one of these four categories can help identify whether it is indeed an ethical issue, not fitting within these categories does not exclude it from being an ethical issue.)

Steps to Approaching Ethical Issues

Many experts have suggested formats to use when approaching an ethical issue. Jameton (1984) describes the following helpful six-step approach:

1. **Identify the problem:** State the problem or the cause of the conflict as clearly as you can.

2. **Gather data:** What information helps to describe or clarify the problem? What information is needed? This information might include history of the problem, the patient's or family's situation and views or wishes, or legal or administrative considerations.

3. **Identify options:** What courses of action are available to take? What are the probable outcomes? What are the short-term and long-term consequences?

4. **Think the ethical problem through:** Determine what the most important issue of the case is. This often helps guide the course of action.

5. **Make a decision:** Decide on the course of action most appropriate for the case and most consistent with personal judgments and ethical beliefs, taking into account judgments made by colleagues involved in the case or with whom the case has been discussed. Also consider the professional values and ethics of nursing practice and, more specifically, of critical care. The American Nurses Association (2001) and the AACN (2010) discuss nursing's obligations to patients and society in their published Code of Ethics documents. These are both readily available for nurses to refer to and to help guide their practice.

6. **Act and assess:** Proceed down the chosen route. After doing so, assess the outcome and results. Were the expected or desired outcomes achieved? How do the outcomes differ from the desired outcomes? What can be done differently next time? Are you satisfied with the outcome?

Unfortunately, the outcome that occurs is not always the outcome nurses desire. Though taking action and attempting to resolve the ethical problem(s) can further help nurses in advocating for the patient and reconciling their personal ethical beliefs with their professional obligations, they might need to take additional steps, such as personal counseling or debriefing sessions. Also, when nurses are going through the steps in actuality, they might notice many of the steps appear to be combined. This reality is exemplified in the two case studies discussed later in this chapter.

What Avenues Are Available to Help?

Different hospitals and health-related systems of care offer different resources for addressing ethical problems. Nurses will find it best to know what options are readily available should an ethical problem arise. However, if a problem arises and nurses are unsure of their available options, a human resources representative or the unit manager can often help point nurses in the right direction. See Table 8.2 for possible options in addressing ethical issues.

Table 8.2   Addressing Ethical Issues

	Possible Options	Whom to Approach If Options Are Unknown
Ethics Resources	-Ethics Consultation -Ethics Hotline -Ethics Mediation	-Human Resources -Unit Manager -Clinical Nurse Specialist
Personal Resources	-Personal Counseling -Clergy -Counselor	
Team Approaches	-Time Outs -Grief Rounds -Debriefing Sessions	

During hospital orientation programs, the hospital usually attempts to familiarize nurses with the available options. Typically, any member of the health care team can call for an ethics consult by an ethicist. Although not every institution allows anonymous calling, some anonymous ethics hotlines are available for discussing or reporting a problem. These avenues typically help nurses work through the problem and provide various solutions or alternative options available. If mediation is available, meetings between the parties involved can help make the issues clearer and bring all involved parties together to attempt to resolve the problem.

In other circumstances, personal counseling for nurses might be a more appropriate avenue to take. For example, if a situation occurred where nurses felt they were unable to intervene appropriately and were now trying to cope with the consequences of the unethical actions, or if nurses were able to act on a problem but could not achieve the desired outcome, they could call a clergy member or a counselor within the hospital (if available) to discuss or debrief. This can help nurses verbalize their concerns and feelings and cope with the situation at hand. Often, time outs, grief rounds, or debriefing sessions are helpful for the team members involved in particularly stressful situations, including deaths. Specifically, time outs provide a forum for the interdisciplinary team to meet within 24 hours after a patient's death to discuss feelings regarding the situation (Richmond & Craig, 1985), and grief rounds allow the interdisciplinary team to meet every few weeks to discuss concerns in an open, inviting manner (Abrahm, 2005). These avenues can be helpful for nurses and other health care professionals to discuss their feelings or any problematic issues and possibly devise solutions to commonly occurring problems.

AACN has published a handbook to help critical-care nurses confront and deal with moral distress (Rushton & Westphal, 2004). Their handbook suggests that when nurses are confronted with problems related to a patient situation, involving the family in patient care is highly recommended. Encouraging family members to ask questions, giving them avenues for hands-on care, and keeping them informed of the patient's status can help keep the family on board with the care provided. Additionally, the AACN suggests that using outside services, such as ethics committees, social work, palliative care, and chaplains, not only helps nurses advocate for the patient and family but also keeps everyone focused on the goals of patient care. Identifying leadership within the unit to help handle the situation, such as a nurse manager, clinical nurse specialist, or coworker with ethics experience, would also be valuable. In addition, creating an ongoing support group or mentorship program within the unit is helpful for nurses to discuss similar situations or other situations causing them distress.

If an issue arises within the health care team, AACN recommends further avenues to conquer these issues (Rushton & Westphal, 2004). AACN suggests that nurses should be clear about their desire to collaborate with the other party involved by attending rounds, listening, and taking responsibility for their actions. Carefully assessing their responses to members of the health care team to avoid projecting negative experiences or feelings can help facilitate collaboration on their part; it also projects the appearance of assuming that other providers desire collaboration as well.

Nurses can also facilitate collaboration by attempting to provide continuity of care between providers and by seeking out formal mechanisms for conflict resolution, including ethics committees and patient/family representatives. Finally, personally addressing the individual contributing to a nurse's distress with assertive, nonemotional statements can help begin a dialogue about the problem. For example, if nurses feel that the physician is providing a patient's family with false hope, they might use the following statement to begin a dialogue with the physician: "Mr. Gray continues to have unstable vital signs. In rounds, we have discussed with the team that his likelihood for survival is small. Mr. Gray's wife does not seem to understand this. How can we help her understand this better?"

Hospitals often have specific procedures in place for calling attention to or dealing with some types of ethical issues. However, even if no specific resources are available institutionally, nurses can take actions to confront and deal with the issue at hand. The critical-care case studies that follow exemplify how nurses can confront ethical issues in two different situations in two alternate manners.

Case Study 8.2

A 65-year-old woman is hospitalized with a long history of chronic obstructive pulmonary disease and metastatic lung cancer to the breast, spine, and brain. She has been hospitalized for 3 months and has had a total of 25 surgeries. Currently, she has a tracheostomy and is mechanically ventilated. Because of her pulmonary status, she has been unable to wean from the ventilator. The nurses' documentation of neurological assessments states that the patient is alert and oriented. Although she goes in and out of consciousness and has only weak motor control, she is able to communicate by nodding her head and pointing on an alphabet chart.

At this time, the patient has developed a subdural hematoma requiring another surgery. The patient communicates to the husband and nurse, saying, "Stop. No more. You're hurting me. This is killing me." The nurse communicates this information to the health care team. The physicians respond to the patient by telling her, "No, you need these surgeries to live." The nurse feels the physician is giving the husband misleading information to sway his decision to continue care. The husband loves his wife and is clinging to any words of hope; he wants her to live at any cost and goes along with what the physician explains as necessary. The nurse is in the room when the physician explains to the husband that the patient has been sick for a long time and is probably confused and unable to make "those kinds of decisions." The nurse sees the patient turn to her, which the nurse interprets as asking for help. The nurse speaks up and says to the husband and the physician that in her assessments, the patient is oriented and understands the situation and clearly expresses her desire to stop.

When the nurse and physician leave the room, the physician is upset with her for not supporting him while speaking with the patient's family and believes the nurse acted out of line.

1. Assess the situation. Identify the problem.

To proceed, the nurse first needs to assess the situation. Is she feeling conflicted? Yes. Why, though? What are the problems in play? The nurse feels trapped between advocating for what the patient has expressed and what the physicians are communicating to the patient and her family. While the nurses are documenting that the patient is alert and oriented, what is her state of mind to make these types of decisions? Is the husband acting out of the best interests of the patient, or is he acting on his own interests? In whose interest is the physician acting?

The nurse feels as though she is being asked to act against the patient's will. While assessing the situation, she attempts to keep the family informed of the patient's status, and she encourages the husband to ask questions and participate in the patient's care so he can get a clear idea of her mental capacity. However, the nurse feels that the husband is grasping onto any hopeful words, and that each time the physician speaks to him, the physician gives him false hope.

After assessing the situation, the nurse identifies the main problems as 1) lack of respect for the patient's autonomy, 2) the physician providing misleading information, and 3) conflict between nurse and physician.

2. Gather data.

Next, the nurse needs to describe the situation with pertinent details, excluding irrelevant details. The nurse could suggest a psychological evaluation to assess the patient's state of mind—to determine her mental clarity, whether she is depressed, or whether she has proper decision-making capacity. Furthermore, the nurse can discuss the problem with coworkers for validation and to help clarify the important points.

3. Identify the options and think the ethical problem through.

In this situation, the nurse has several routes she can take. She can talk to her nurse manager to see if there is a policy for handling similar situations on the unit or to see if the manager has suggestions for a resolution. Depending on what is readily available within her hospital, she can seek advice from the ethics committee, the ethics hotline, or department of bioethics, or she can arrange an ethics consult. Alternatively, she can call social work, the hospital chaplain, or another clergy member to speak with her, the patient, and family to try to resolve the situation. In addition, if possible, she can call upon patient/family representatives, who are typically employed by the hospital and work with the family and patient to advocate for their needs and help address their concerns. A consult from the palliative care team might be beneficial as well, as the team can talk with the husband and patient about the options available to them.

4. Make a decision and act.

The nurse makes the decision to call the ethics committee, and an ethicist is sent in to assess the situation. The consultant talks with the nurse, the husband, the patient, and the physician. The recommendation is to get a psychological evaluation to formally assess her capacity for decision-making. A meeting is set up with the physicians, the nurses, and the family so that everyone can have access to the same information and discuss the situation together calmly. However, before the evaluation and meeting can take place, the husband decides to consent to the surgery, and the patient undergoes the procedure recommended by the physician. Despite this, the ethics consultant ultimately determines that the patient does have capacity to make decisions and that her wishes should be followed. An additional meeting is held with the physicians, nurses, family, and ethics consultant, and the husband begins to understand and accept the situation. Ultimately, the patient undergoes no additional surgeries, the palliative care team is called, and the patient passes away quietly.

5. Assess.

In assessing the situation, the nurse must compare the resulting outcome with her desired outcome. She also must reflect and determine her resulting feelings about the situation. Although the nurse ultimately felt she did the right thing for the patient, initially she felt very angry when the patient underwent her last surgery. However, as the process continued, she began to feel better and felt as though she was advocating for her patient in the best way that she could. Alternatively, if the nurse had not had formal ethics routes available to her, she could have gained support from her colleagues and continued to speak with the physicians and family until she felt she had adequately advocated for her patient.

If the nurse continues to feel that the problem was not resolved adequately or she still feels distressed, the hospital might have a counselor she can speak with to try to work out her feelings. Alternatively, a support group might be available for the nurse to join. Discussing and resolving her feelings can help protect her from potential moral distress and its consequences. Additionally, it can often be helpful to bring the team together retrospectively to discuss the feelings and what could be done differently next time (Richmond & Craig, 1985).

Case Study 8.3

A 32-year-old male comes into the emergency department after sustaining multiple gunshot wounds, with at least one to the left side of his chest. The patient had been intubated in the field, and his vital signs remain unstable in the emergency department after initial resuscitation efforts. After the resuscitation begins, the nurse feels the trauma team has made the decision that the patient's injuries were not compatible with life. She feels the consensus was that the team would not be able to repair the injuries in the trauma bay and that he would not survive to make it to the operating room.

Contrary to what the nurse feels the team has decided about the patient's survivability, the physicians decide to open his chest in an attempt to stop the bleeding. They are able to visualize the injury to the aorta and the subclavian artery, affirming that the injury is not a survivable injury. The physicians then proceed to insert a Foley catheter and inflate it to tamponade the bleeding. The nurse has never seen this attempted and feels that the physicians are "grasping at straws." The resuscitation efforts continue. The trauma team continues to open more sterile packages, procedure kits and intravenous lines and to give more and more blood and intravenous fluids. The nurse looks around and sees "gallons" of blood on the floor—all blood that she had been responsible for administering. She feels that she and the team are wasting resources when the decision has already been made that the injury was unsurvivable.

The nurse is conflicted because she feels other patients could be using these resources and benefitting from them. The nurse is frustrated with the situation. She feels that every patient deserves the team's best efforts, but if the decision has been made that the injury is not survivable, she wonders, "What are we doing?"

---

1. Assess the situation. Identify the problem.

Emergency situations can take place in many locations, including not only the emergency department, but also the critical-care unit. Inherently, ethical problems in emergent situations are more difficult to work through, because the atmosphere is fast-paced, people move quickly, and decisions must be made with little time for deliberation. However, the nurse still needs to assess the problem quickly and decide whether she will act on the problem, and if so, when—now or after the situation is over.

First, clearly, the nurse is feeling conflicted. She feels conflicted over using finite and expensive resources on a patient that she feels (and thought the trauma team agreed) would very likely not benefit. Because she does feel that other patients would benefit from those resources, her ethical problem is a resource allocation issue, or, more broadly, a justice issue. She also has mixed feelings as to the goals of the resuscitation and questions the utility of continuing treatment.

2. Gather data.

The nurse quickly attempts to gather information mentally about the situation. She recognizes that the patient is young with no significant medical history, making the recovery odds slightly better, but she sees the patient's extensive injuries and recalls the trauma team agreeing that the patient would not survive these injuries and that there was not much they could do to treat him. She also sees that the trauma team seems intent on continuing the resuscitation.

3. Identify the options and think the ethical problem through.

In the heat of a fast-paced situation, the nurse must quickly sort out her options. Some options in the preceding case include voicing her concern immediately, in hopes of changing the course of the resuscitation; further assessing the problem after the resuscitation is over, acknowledging that this is a recurrent issue that needs to be addressed; and discussing the problem after the resuscitation with a wider audience, including her nurse manager, the trauma team, and ethics consultants.

4. Make a decision and act.

During the resuscitation, the nurse feels uncomfortable speaking up about stopping resuscitative efforts and wasting resources. She feels that with so many people and opinions in the room, her opinions would not really be heard. She continues to follow the physicians' orders and participate in attempting to resuscitate the patient. Ultimately, the patient does not survive. When the resuscitation is over, she opts to share her feelings with the nurse manager about the way the resuscitation took place. She had been involved with other resuscitations where she had felt similarly and knew that other nurses felt the same way. The nurse and her manager decide to call a debriefing session to talk about how the resuscitation was run and how similar situations should be handled in the future. They invite an ethicist from the ethics committee to the debriefing for an outside prospective. The meeting runs smoothly, and the participants decide that a policy should be written for the department on how to manage situations where the trauma team is certain that the patient's injuries are not compatible with life.

 PURPOSE EXERCISE: CONSIDER AND WRITE YOUR ANSWERS TO THE FOLLOWING QUESTIONS

1. In the past, when you were ethically opposed to what was occurring with a patient, did you stop and discuss it then or at another time?

2. Would you act in the same manner in the future?

5. Assess.

In assessing the situation, the nurse feels content with the way she acted and the results that occurred. Her desired outcome matched well with the resulting outcome. In hindsight, though, she feels that it might have been possible to voice her concern during the resuscitation, while being prepared not to push the issue further if her vocalization was not well received. She does recognize that discussing ethical issues in emergent situations is often difficult, and that speaking up about such issues is likely to be met with resistance. However, she decides that she will attempt it in the future anyway.

- If you were this nurse, would you feel comfortable confronting the issue during the resuscitation, or would you deal with it after the resuscitation had concluded?

- With whom would you initially discuss the issue?

Both of these case studies differ in scenario and location, but they are clear examples of the kinds of ethical issues frequently encountered by critical-care nurses. Both nurses were able to identify the main issues and what their options were, and act accordingly. Having multiple options available to deal with ethical problems enables nurses to choose an appropriate course of action they feel comfortable with to confront the problem.

Conclusion

Though the steps proposed to assist nurses address ethical challenges in clinical practice are helpful and outline specific steps to work through any given ethical problem, they are not precise. But to appropriately care for critically ill patients, nurses need to be able to advocate for their patients' needs, collaborate with colleagues, and reconcile their own personal values while working within the health care system. Today's critical-care nurses need to be equipped to tackle not only physiological and psychological problems, but ethical problems as well.

Recognizing the ethical issue you are experiencing is important. If you are feeling conflicted over a patient care issue that is related to a value, moral, or ethic, you are experiencing an ethical issue:

- Consider how to approach ethical issues and what avenues are available to you within your unit and within your hospital. Familiarizing yourself with these before experiencing ethical issues is beneficial.

- Decide how you are going to deal with the issue and act on it.

- Remember to assess and reflect on how the issue was dealt with and how you ultimately feel about the situation.

Talk About It!

- Consider a situation you might experience that could cause you to have moral distress. Discuss this with a nonjudgmental colleague or friend and formulate a plan about how to handle the situation if it ever arises.

- Consider how your critical-care unit approaches ethical issues. Are you comfortable navigating the system? What about your colleagues. Talk about it with your colleagues and talk about what steps you can individually, and as a team, take to increase your comfort in confronting issues when they arise?

- Consider a specific patient encounter you have had that caused you to feel ethically conflicted. How were you affected by this? What did you do about the situation? What would you do now? What specific avenues would you take and who would you recruit to help with the situation? Explore this issue with your colleagues. Each of you will have a different encounter that can help prepare the others for potentially difficult situations in the future.

References

Abrahm, J. L. (2005). *A physician's guide to pain and symptom management in cancer patients* (2nd ed.). Baltimore: Johns Hopkins University Press.

Alt-White, A. C., & Pranulis, M. F. (2006). Addressing nurses' ethical concerns about research in critical care settings. *Nursing Administration Quarterly, 30*(1), 67-75.

American Association of Critical-Care Nurses (AACN). (2004). *Moral distress position statement.* Aliso Viejo, CA: Author.

American Association of Critical-Care Nurses (AACN). (2010). *Key statements, beliefs, and philosophies behind the American Association of Critical-Care Nurses.* Retrieved from http://www.aacn.org/WD/Memberships/Content/Mission_vision_values_ethics.pcms?menu=AboutUs#ethic

American Nurses Association. (2001). *Code of ethics for nurses with interpretive statements.* Retrieved from http://www.nursingworld.org/MainMenuCategories/EthicsStandards/CodeofEthicsforNurses.aspx

Beauchamp, T. L., & Childress, J. F. (2001). *Principles of biomedical ethics* (5th ed.). Oxford, UK: Oxford University Press.

Fry, S. T., Harvey, R. M., Hurley, A. C., & Foley, B. J. (2002). Development of a model of moral distress in military nursing. *Nursing Ethics: An International Journal for Health Care Professionals, 9*(4), 373-387.

Holly, C. M. (1993). The ethical quandaries of acute care nursing practice. *Journal of Professional Nursing, 9*(2), 110-115.

Hough, M. C. (2008). Learning, decisions and transformation in critical care nursing practice. *Nursing Ethics, 15*(3), 322-331.

Jameton, A. (1984). *Nursing practice: The ethical issues.* Englewood Cliffs, NJ: Prentice-Hall Inc.

Kelly, B. (1998). Preserving moral integrity: A follow-up study with new graduate nurses. *Journal of Advanced Nursing, 28*(5), 1134-1145.

Meltzer, L. S., & Huckabay, L. M. (2004). Critical care nurses' perceptions of futile care and its effect on burnout. *American Journal of Critical Care, 13*(3), 202-208.

Raines, M. L. (2000). Ethical decisions making in nurses: Relationships among moral reasoning, coping style, and ethics stress. *JONAS Healthcare Law, Ethics, & Regulation, 2*(1), 29-41.

Redman, B. K., & Fry, S. T. (2000). Nurses' ethical conflicts: What is really known about them? *Nursing Ethics: An International Journal for Health Care Professionals, 7*(4), 360-366.

Richmond, T., & Craig, M. (1985). Timeout: Facing death in the ICU. *Dimensions in Critical Care Nursing, 4*(1), 41-45.

Richmond, T. S., & Ulrich, C. (2007). Ethical issues of recruitment and enrollment of critically ill and injured patients for research. *AACN Advanced Critical Care, 18*(4), 352-355.

Rushton, C. H., & Westphal, C. G. (2004). *The 4A's to rise above moral distress handbook.* American Association of Critical Care Nurses. Retrieved http://www.aacn.org/WD/Practice/Docs/4As_to_Rise_Above_Moral_Distress.pdf

Ulrich, C. M., Hamric, A. B, & Grady, C. (2010). Moral distress: A growing problem in the health professions? *Hastings Center Report, 40*(1), 20-22.

Viney, C. (1996). A phenomenological study of ethical decision-making among senior intensive care nurses and doctors concerning withdrawal of treatment. *Nursing in Critical Care, 1*(4), 182-187.

Wilkinson, J. M. (1988). Moral distress in nursing practice: Experience and effect. *Nursing Forum, 23*(1), 16-29.

Zeitzer, M. B. (2010). Ethical issues and decision making related to resuscitation of severely injured patients: Perceptions of emergency department nurses. *Dissertation Abstract International, 70*(10). UMI No. AAT 3381887.

ETHICS IN LONG-TERM CARE 9

–Michele Mathes, JD
Education Director
Center for Advocacy for the Rights and
Interests of the Elderly

Think About It!

- The nature of long-term care presents nurses with unique ethical challenges.

- The particular nature and challenges of long-term care call for the application of a distinctive ethical framework.

- An ethical framework based upon commitment to the care recipient best captures the responsibilities of nurses working in long-term care settings.

- The responsibilities of long-term care providers are comprised within five overarching commitments to care recipients.

- The *IDEAS* decision-making process offers a pathway for resolving ethical dilemmas when they arise.

History reflects our evolving understanding about the proper goals of long-term care and the kind of care to which frail older adults are entitled. Today, possibly more than at any time in our past, the purposes of long-term care are being deeply examined, debated, and discussed. Resulting changes in policy and practice, though generally welcomed, pose new ethical challenges for practitioners in the field. This chapter presents an ethics of responsibility approach to addressing ethical issues that arise in the course of providing long-term care.

Long-term care settings offer both unique opportunities and unique challenges for nurses. One significant opportunity is the opportunity to exercise greater professional autonomy than is the norm in most acute care settings. Although nursing homes are required to have medical directors, their responsibilities are largely administrative and supervisory. Medical directors are often part-time, serving in that role at several nursing home facilities. In most cases, the medical director is not involved in the routine medical care of individual residents; rather, they have oversight responsibility for the quality of clinical care. Responsibility for individual residents' medical care generally lies with their attending physicians, whose visits might be (and very often are) sporadic and perfunctory. Thus, nursing staff carry the responsibility for the day-to-day management of the health care, and health, of residents. This chapter proposes a new approach to understanding the ethical foundations of long-term care in terms of the commitments that care providers make to the recipients of their care. It has benefitted from input from long-term care providers at every stage of its development. The framework presented reflects both the changing role of long-term care and the experience of those working in the field.

Working in long-term care brings unique challenges as well. These challenges arise from both the nature of long-term care and the vulnerability of the individuals who are the recipients of care, a significant proportion of whom have some degree of cognitive impairment. In recent years, increased attention has been given to providing the services and supports needed to enable older adults to continue to live in their homes and communities as long as possible. Thus, those who move to residential facilities on a long-term basis are often very frail—for example, elders who have some degree of dementia or other mental impairment and are in need of around-the-clock supervision and those with the most extensive ongoing health care needs.

As our concepts about and goals for long-term care have developed, recognition of the importance of understanding long-term care facilities as residents' *homes* has increased. Hearing long-term care staff, especially direct care staff who have the day-to-day responsibility for hands-on care of residents, say that "we are their family" is quite common. Daily personal care, getting to know a resident's family, living through holidays and occasions, celebration, and suffering all create the possibility for intimate connection with those for whom care is provided. Those who see this possibility as an opportunity will find long-term care professionally and personally deeply gratifying.

Case Study 9.1

Mrs. Hanson, 83, has Alzheimer's-type dementia, severe osteoarthritis, type II diabetes mellitus, and has been a resident of the Green Bower Nursing Home for 5 years. For many years before that, Mrs. Hanson lived with her daughter and son-in-law, but as her mobility decreased, caring for her became exceedingly difficult. Five years ago, Mrs. Hanson's children reluctantly admitted her to the nursing home. She had not completed an advance directive prior to admission and was believed to lack the capacity legally required to complete one at the time of admission.

About 9 months ago, Mrs. Hanson developed chronic renal failure. She began receiving hemodialysis for which she was taken out to a dialysis center 3 days a week. Despite her dementia, her daughter and physician observed that she had a reasonably good quality of life, enjoyed a variety of activities in the nursing home, and tolerated the dialysis well.

Over the past 5 months, however, Mrs. Hanson's cognitive ability has declined markedly. Now, she only occasionally recognizes her daughter and is entirely dependent for her activities of daily living. Although she is mostly mute, she does seem to experience pleasure when being spoon-fed or when listening to an accordion player who visits the home regularly. Throughout this time, her daughter has continued to visit frequently and has always appeared to have her mother's best interests in mind.

In the past month, each trip to dialysis has become an ordeal. Mrs. Hanson resists getting on the transport gurney and fights the introduction of arteriovenous catheters. A medical workup reveals no new underlying illness to account for this change in behavior, and her physician ascribes her response to progressive dementia. Some members of the nursing staff are beginning to believe that dialysis is more of a burden than a benefit for Mrs. Hanson. They believe it should be discontinued, and Mrs. Hanson should be allowed to die peacefully.

Without dialysis, Mrs. Hanson would surely die within a couple of weeks. The nursing home administrator and director of nursing discuss the situation with Mrs. Hanson's daughter, who insists that her mother continue to receive dialysis. She argues that "mom has always had a strong spirit and would want to live every day the Lord gives her" and that she deserves to have "everything" done for her. The staff of Green Bower are divided. Though some staff believe that continuing dialysis is causing Mrs. Hanson to suffer needlessly and that transferring her to the hospice unit of the nursing home is appropriate at this point, other staff members, especially the direct care staff who have provided the daily hands-on care for Mrs. Hanson and have become very attached to her, are deeply distressed at the thought that Green Bower will simply stop sending her for dialysis. They believe that it's wrong to withdraw this life-sustaining treatment from her when her health status hasn't declined significantly. The administrator and the director of nursing decide to call a team meeting of the staff involved in Mrs. Hanson's care.

The Nature of Long-Term Care

Long-term care is profoundly different from acute care. Virtually every aspect of a resident's experience is shaped by life in a nursing home. Thus, though acute care focuses primarily on discrete medical problems, nursing homes are charged with responsibility for the "global" well-being of care recipients, including their emotional, spiritual, psychological, and social well-being, as well as physical health.

Second, though the exclusivity of the doctor-patient relationship is a strongly held traditional value in acute care medicine, in long-term care much value is given to a resident's place within a web of relationships with family members and friends. The importance these relationships hold for her or his emotional well-being cannot be overstated. Strategies that support and strengthen these relationships rather than create barriers to participation in care by loved ones are encouraged.

A third difference between acute and long-term care is the nature of the involvement between long-term care staff and care recipients, which is daily, continual, and ongoing for months and years.

Fourth, prevailing models of medical ethics start with an understanding of the relationship between doctor and patient as one between independent and autonomous agents. Decision-making is believed to rest ultimately with the patient, although a collaborative relationship is often regarded as the ideal. The reality of long-term care is quite different. Care recipients most often are physically frail and/or suffer from various forms of dementia and other cognitive impairments. In facility-based care, the experience of dependency is magnified by the sheer variety of ways in which the quality of the resident's daily life is reliant upon facility staff. A model of decision-making predicated on the autonomy of the care recipient does not reflect the reality of long-term care settings.

Finally, unlike in acute care where, historically at least, the interests of individual patients do not compete with each other, in long-term care the needs or wishes of one resident might be in conflict with the needs or wishes of other residents. Thus, residents' interests and rights need to be balanced against one another.

Though notions of "right" and "wrong" might be written into our genetic code, how to discern one from the other continues to challenge philosophers and theologians. This is probably most true in the health care fields. For approximately a century, the law has recognized the right of a patient who has the mental capacity needed to make a medical decision to make that decision and the obligation of the health care provider to defer to that decision. This right has subsequently become well-established in medical ethics as well (Beauchamp & Childress, 2008). However, professionals, whether in medicine or many other fields, come into relationship with those whom they care for or serve with their own professional ethical obligations. If professionals are to be moral agents rather than simply service vendors, decision-making needs to take account of these professionals' ethical obligations as well.

Margaret Urban Walker has written of an "ethics of responsibility" (Walker, 1997). The basic idea of it is that we are responsible to those who are vulnerable to our actions. The vulnerability that creates moral responsibility in another might arise in three ways, according to Walker. The first way is through the nature of the relationship between the persons involved. Relationships of parents and children, husbands and wives, friends, or partners create mutual vulnerabilities through the feelings of love, trust, and dependence. By entering into and remaining within such a relationship with another person, we become responsible in some way to the other in whom we have implicitly allowed such feelings to develop.

The second way another person becomes vulnerable to us so that we are responsible to him or her is through our making explicit representations upon which the other is permitted or encouraged to rely. For example, if we expressly tell someone that she can depend upon us for certain things, if we say we will be true to another, if we promise to stand by a friend, that person becomes vulnerable, physically and/or emotionally, to our carrying through on what we said. Therefore, we have become morally responsible to her or him.

Walker also proposes that one person becomes responsible to another through the extreme plight of the one and the unique ability or proximity of the other to provide assistance. Thus, we recognize the moral responsibility of an adult who is able to swim to save a drowning child, even if that child is a stranger to him.

The "ethics of responsibility" Walker proposes provides a basis for long-term care providers' moral responsibility to the recipients of their care. The very nature of the caregiving relationship gives rise to reliance and trust in the care receiver. "I will take care of you" is the implicit and explicit pledge of a long-term care professional. In addition, care providers encourage care receivers to engage them by specifying the kinds and quality of care they provide, which in turn leads others to make choices about whom they will entrust with the care of themselves or their loved ones. Thus, the ethics of responsibility takes account of both the particular professional obligations of the care provider and the particular vulnerability of the care recipient within the long-term care setting.

Developing an Ethical Framework for Long-Term Care

Understanding that this combination of professional obligation and care-recipient vulnerability leads to long-term care providers being morally responsible to care receivers *in some way*, we now need to figure out the nature and parameters of their responsibilities. Mathes and Menio in *Competence with Compassion: Ethical Choices in Long-Term Services and Supports* (2007) propose that the responsibilities of long-term care providers fall within five themes. These overarching themes reflect the broad commitments that long-term care providers implicitly make to care recipients and are identified as the foundational ethical obligations of long-term care providers:

- Respect and support residents' self-determination

- Recognize and provide opportunity for the continuation of their individual life story

- Preserve and promote their health

- Protect their safety

- Ease their suffering and pain

Although each professional and staff member within a long-term care organization will have her or his respective areas of expertise, each staff person, as well as the organization as a whole, assumes responsibility for the fulfillment of these five commitments.

The Commitment to Respect and Support Self-Determination

As previously noted, "respect for autonomy," understood as the obligation to defer to a mentally capacitated individual's decisions, is a well-established principle of clinical ethics. The substitution of "self-determination" for "autonomy" in the *Competence with Compassion* framework is both intentional and significant.

The concept of human autonomy originated at a specific time and place: Europe in the 18th century. For thousands of years before that, and even today in cultures other than those with Western European cultural roots, the concept of an autonomous person was unknown or even nonsensical. The idea of human autonomy developed in response to the great leaps in scientific knowledge experienced during the period known as the Enlightenment and the great value given to scientific (that is, rational) thought. Humans' ability to think rationally was offered as the basis for our autonomy, that is, our ability to make deliberative decisions for ourselves. The same historical period also gave birth to American and French revolutionary cries for liberty. To these intellectual movements that emphasize rationality and freedom, add the American commitment to individualism born of pioneer and frontier life, and it is not difficult to understand the central role the notion of autonomy plays in our social, political, and psychological heritage.

Two important observations we can take from the preceding information are these:

1. Human beings have not been, and are not now, universally or eternally understood to be autonomous; to the contrary, the idea of a "personal autonomy" is time and culture bound.

2. A capacity for rational thinking is the lynchpin of personal autonomy; that is, without the ability to reason, the very idea of autonomy falls apart.

The recognition that autonomy is not necessary to and inherent in being human, that other people in other places and other times understand being "human" differently, opens the possibility of examining the concept of autonomy to see what it holds of value for us.

What does it mean to be autonomous? Words commonly used to define the term are *independent* and *self-reliant*. The *Oxford Advanced Learner Dictionary* gives the sense of the word *autonomous* as "able to do things and make decisions without help from anyone else." Autonomous decisions are accorded great respect and deference because they reflect individualism, reason, and liberty, each a deeply held and abiding cultural value.

If we acknowledge that we can be human beings and deserving of respect on bases other than our autonomy, then we might begin to ask whether holding up autonomy as a primary ethical value actually serves us, or whether privileging other concepts (for example, community, connection, interdependence) might better serve our interests and needs. The fact that ability to reason is necessary to any meaningful understanding of autonomy should move us to question the ethical centrality given to autonomous decision-making. The description of autonomous decision-making does not fit many of the frail elders who live in long-term care facilities, who must rely on others to meet many of their most basic and intimate needs, and who suffer with various degrees of cognitive impairment. However, notwithstanding this lack of "fit" between the actual meaning of autonomy and the reality of vulnerable elders' lives, we are reluctant to give up the language of autonomy, because we recognize that the concept itself does hold within it something that we believe to be extremely important and valuable.

The notion of human autonomy implicitly, if not explicitly, speaks to the existence of boundaries between persons that both legally and ethically must not be breached. We generally understand that the right to privacy in one's thoughts and actions and the right to be let alone are basic to human dignity. However, long-term care residents, having left their connections in the communities that they came from, including their relationships with neighbors, shopkeepers, church, and community organizations that might have been built over decades or even a lifetime, also need the opportunity for forging connection. Despite the cultural and historical importance accorded to individualism in the United States, we know that the development and sustaining of a healthy sense of oneself, indeed the very sense of *being* a self, are dependent upon our being in relationship with others. To the extent that respecting autonomy entails taking a "hands off" stance, it discourages the very sort of engagement that might support nursing home residents, psychologically and physically. Perhaps, then, another concept can incorporate the aspects of autonomy we value, but not suggest the separation that might challenge other values of ethical importance in the care of frail elders.

We propose that the language of autonomy be replaced by that of self-determination. This is understood as the *determination of one's own fate or course of action without compulsion* (Self-determination, n.d.). Deference to decisions that are arrived at based upon an understanding of the relevant facts and alternatives and that reflect a consistent set of values is warranted both legally and ethically. Such deference fulfills both an ethical commitment to respect self-determination and the legal requirement for informed consent. However, by deemphasizing independence, respect for self-determination leaves open the possibility of offering support and collaboration in the decision-making process to enhance the ability of frail elders, including those with compromised capacity, to make decisions for themselves and for their futures.

Respecting and supporting self-determination require us to be attentive to more than just the decisions made and articulated by care recipients. Making decisions for oneself is only a part of what being self-determining means. In addition to the decisions we make and communicate, how we constitute our self might be expressed verbally or nonverbally, through the values we live and the goals we have sought to achieve.

Our daily experience makes us keenly aware that a whole person comprises more than cognitive skills. We are also emotional and creative beings. In addition, many, if not most, people believe that human beings have a spiritual dimension as well. A significant number of long-term care recipients do not have the capacity to make decisions that meet the traditional criteria for being considered "reasoned" and, therefore, autonomous. They might no longer be able to formulate goals for themselves. They might not be able to state a coherent set of values that they can use to sort through options. They might not be able to understand the potential consequences of their choices, for themselves, or for others. Even so, they certainly might have preferences for what they want to do and might express these preferences very clearly in words or in actions.

In some situations, care receivers lose the ability to express preferences as well as decisions. Respecting and supporting self-determination when a care recipient lacks the capacity to express a preference might include making care choices consistent with prior written and spoken directives by the patient; consulting with surrogate decision-makers chosen by the patient; and being aware of the care recipient's life story as a reflection of values and prior choices, so that nonverbal or inarticulate cues about choices might be better understood.

The Commitment to Enable the Continuation and Completion of the Resident's Life Story

Many, if not most, people anticipate needing long-term care with a sense of dread. In part, the reason for the dread stems from the belief that the need for long-term care, either from intrusive home care providers or through a move to a nursing home, marks the end of one's personal life story. To paraphrase bioethicist James Rachels, the individual's biographical life is over, while his or her biological life goes on (Rachels, 1986).

Too often in health care settings, including long-term care, information about a care receiver comes from sources other than the person herself or himself. Care providers look to medical records, admissions forms, and information from family members for the care recipient's "history," which we take as the medical as well as psychosocial story of who that person was and is. But each of these narrative sources speaks in its particular voice and from its own perspective, reflecting its particular concerns and biases. To care well for individual persons requires that we know them not just as others do, but much more importantly, as each individual knows him/herself.

The value that life narratives hold is not simply as interesting stories, although they certainly may be that. The sidebar on the next page identifies the ways in which knowledge of a resident's life story contributes to the quality of long-term care. Having the opportunity over time to become aware of the older adult's life story and thus to more fully understand the implications of choices and decisions within the context of a life is one of the features of practice in a long-term care setting that most distinguishes it from hospital-based nursing. For those who are drawn to this possibility for deeper relationship with those who need care, long-term care offers special rewards.

> ### The Role of Life Story in Long-Term Care
>
> - It helps maintain self-identity in the face of great change
>
> - It illuminates meanings of events or choices by providing context
>
> - It individualizes care recipients and combats "stereotyping"
>
> - It offers a guide for decision-making when the older adult is not able to make decisions for herself or himself
>
> - It provides social connection between the storyteller and the listener
>
> - It helps exercise, and sustain, memory
>
> - It encourages understanding, empathy, and compassion

The Commitment to Promote and Preserve Health

Most people living in long-term care facilities are there because they suffer with chronic illnesses such as diabetes, arthritis, Parkinson's disease, cancer, congestive heart failure, chronic obstructive pulmonary disease, and/or dementia. One of the most critical areas of health care for nursing home residents is accurate and appropriate medication management. Clearly, highest quality clinical care is of the utmost importance for these most frail elders. However, in light of the prevalence of chronic disease among long-term care residents, the commitment to preserve and promote the resident's health is most often not focused on cure. "Health" in these circumstances relates more to maximizing the resident's functional status than to resolving underlying condition or disease. The commitment to preserve and promote the health of care receivers has a strong focus on how disease and its various treatment options will affect their ability to participate actively in the life, relationships, and activities available to them.

In light of long-term care's focus on the global well-being of the resident, the commitment to preserve and promote the resident's well-being includes providing the resident with full access to any necessary things that will maximize her or his health—a good and medically appropriate diet, adequate sleep, exercise, fresh air, and fulfillment of emotional and psychological needs. An ethically fraught question that long-term care staff confront is the extent to which long-term care providers have responsibility not only for providing those things that are part of a healthy lifestyle, but for preventing unhealthy lifestyle choices by residents. For example, Mrs. Jones is a diabetic, and 2 years ago had her left leg amputated. She routinely asks the dietitian to give her high-carbohydrate, high-sugar snacks and desserts. Maybe Mr. Rimes, an alcoholic, wants to be able to drink in his room, or Miss Miller, who suffers from emphysema, wants a nurse aide to light her cigarette so she can smoke. Ethical dilemmas such as these are extremely challenging for long-term care staff and rarely are resolved "once and for all." However, the five-step *IDEAS* decision-making process, discussed later in this chapter, offers a method for thinking through these difficult care issues.

The Commitment to Protect the Resident's Safety

The commitment to protect the care recipient's safety addresses his or her interaction with the external environment, including the people in that environment. How can the long-term care setting be created or arranged to provide a physically, emotionally, and psychologically safe place for the care recipient to live? This commitment implicates every aspect of care and calls upon every member of the long-term care organization, from housekeeping to dietary, from floor staff to administrative staff. It requires adequate staffing to assure that help is available when needed, whether by residents or by other staff. It means providing adequate and appropriate equipment. It includes assuring that medications and their dosages are accurate, and providing appropriate food in a form that the resident can safely ingest. It means creating an environment where a resident can feel safe emotionally and psychologically, where residents are not afraid of retaliation if they raise concerns, and where they are not abused.

The Commitment to Ease Suffering and Pain

The fifth commitment a long-term care practitioner makes to the persons he or she provides care for is to ease their pain and suffering. Although "pain" and "suffering" are often referred to as if they were a single experience, they are in fact distinct and separable. One might have great pain yet not suffer, or one might have no pain at all yet suffer deeply. Whereas pain is experienced in the body, suffering is emotional or spiritual in nature. The almost universal response to pain is to seek its reduction or, if possible, elimination, but those who suffer might seek to find meaning within the experience of suffering itself. Honoring a commitment to treat a resident's pain and suffering requires awareness of and alertness to the differences between the two, identifying the most appropriate person to provide care (for example, physician, nurse, chaplain, social worker, psychiatrist, psychologist), and recognizing the need for effective intervention in response to these subjective feelings, as much as we do more observable or measurable symptoms.

The Virtues in Long-Term Care

Fully meeting our ethical obligations to frail elders involves not only what we do (that is, fulfilling our commitments) but the qualities of character that inform how we do it. We might respect a person's self-determination by telling her the truth, but we can tell that truth either coldly or compassionately, in a way that hurts or in a way that supports. Virtues, those qualities of character that contribute to living a "good life," are learned through the models we are given. As children, we learned the value of honesty through the story of George Washington and the cherry tree, or Abe Lincoln's walking miles to return a penny. We learned the value of hard work from the story of Horatio Alger. Nelson Mandela offers a model for forgiveness. Mother Teresa served as a model for compassion. Similarly, in long-term care organizations, a culture of virtue is created not through formal education programs so much as through the models provided by the organizational leaders. If administrators demonstrate integrity, are fair, honest, and empathic, then the chances are better that staff will "pay it forward," demonstrating those qualities in their care of residents.

"Ought" Implies "Can"

One ethically challenging situation is that of the "unbefriended" older adult suffering with dementia who lacks both the capacity to make her or his own decisions and a relative or friend able to make those decisions. How can long-term care providers honor their commitments under such circumstances? Ethics does not require us to do the impossible, although "impossible" must not be understood to mean expensive, inconvenient, time-consuming, or problematic. For example, take the case of Mrs. B, an 89-year-old resident with lung cancer with metastases to the brain. She has COPD, CHF, and is beginning to experience kidney failure. To ask whether we should cure Mrs. B. is an ethically empty question, because it is not possible to do. However, to ask whether we should take steps necessary to extend Mrs. B.'s life for 2 weeks or a month (i.e., hydration and dialysis), so that family living at a distance can gather, may have ethical content to the extent it is possible for us to do that. Similarly, if we have no way of learning a resident's story, we cannot provide opportunity and support for the continuation and completion of that story. We might not be able to fulfill a commitment to respect a resident's self-determination if the resident is not able to form or express a choice. Nonetheless, we continue to be bound by the commitments we are able to fulfill, including the preservation and promotion of health, the protection of safety, and the palliation of pain and suffering.

The sidebar below lists the five overarching commitments that long-term care providers make to those for whom they care.

The Five Commitments of Long-Term Care

- Respect and support the resident's self-determination
- Enable the continuation and completion of the resident's life story
- Promote and preserve the resident's health
- Protect the resident's safety
- Ease the resident's suffering and pain

IDEAS for Ethical Decision-Making in Long-Term Care

The commitments discussed above are most often fulfilled naturally in the day-to-day work of long-term care providers. Situations arise, however, and how the commitments of long-term care may be fulfilled is not obvious. In these circumstances, care providers find themselves faced with an ethical dilemma. An ethical dilemma occurs when 1) there are two or more incompatible right courses of action, so that doing one of them precludes doing the other, or 2) when every option has both right and wrong aspects to it. *IDEAS for Ethical Decision-Making in Long-Term Care (IDEAS)* is a process to help work through ethical dilemmas that arise in providing long-term care.

The word *IDEAS* is an acronym; each letter of the word *IDEAS* stands for a step in the decision-making process. The five steps are: 1) Identify the dilemma and the stakeholders; 2) develop the relevant information and the resident narrative; 3) explore all potential options; 4) assess the options; and 5) select a course of action.

Step 1: Identify the Ethical Dilemma and the Stakeholders

It is critical to begin the process of decision-making by clearly identifying the ethical dilemma to be resolved. This will permit those involved in problem-solving, whether it's a single individual or a team, to "keep their eye on the ball." Ethics lends itself to wide-ranging discussions, while health care generally requires action-focused decisions. Specifying the dilemmas provides a focus point for discussion and helps define the outcome that is needed from the discussion.

Within the ethics framework presented in this chapter, an ethical dilemma is understood as tension between two or more of the long-term care provider's commitments to the recipient of care, i.e., when fulfilling one commitment appears to be incompatible with fulfilling one or more of the remaining commitments. Step 1 of the *IDEAS* process is to identify which commitments are in tension in the issue at hand. Often, staff tend to identify the ethical dilemma in terms of the facts or behavior related to the care receiver at the center of the situation. For example, the perceived dilemma may be stated as "Mrs. Gorman wants to go for walks alone off the nursing home premises, even though her mobility is limited and she often falls," or "Mr. Johnson refuses to get out of bed," or "Miss Ridge doesn't have capacity and doesn't have an advance directive." These facts give rise to ethical dilemmas but are not themselves dilemmas. They present ethical dilemmas because these cases confront care providers with a conflict among their commitments to each resident. In the case of Mrs. Gorman, the conflict is between the commitments to respect her self-determination and the continuation of her life story (she has taken an afternoon walk by herself every afternoon for the past 40 years) on the one hand, and a commitment to preserve her safety on the other. Regarding Mr. Johnson, the dilemma arises from the conflict between the commitments to respect his self-determination and to preserve and promote his health. In the third situation, the dilemma would appear to arise from questions about how to fulfill the commitments to Miss Ridge at the end of life.

Defining an ethical dilemma in terms of the commitments of the care provider rather than in terms of facts about the care recipient makes resolution possible. We might never be able to change Mrs. Gorman's desire to go for walks in the community, or Mr. Johnson's insistence on staying in bed, or know what Miss Ridge's end-of-life choices would have been. What we can do is address our conflicting commitments using an organized process of analysis.

The *IDEAS* process is resident-centered, and the ethical dilemma is resolved in terms of the commitments to the resident. However, the process should include an awareness of the concerns of others, such as staff or family who also might have significant interests at stake. A full resolution of the dilemma should address the concerns expressed by other stakeholders in some way (for example, with education or training, grief counseling, dispute resolution, peer discussion groups, etc.).

Step 2: Develop the Relevant Information and the Resident Narrative

To the extent that residents can participate in the decision-making process, we need to listen to them, to the preferences, values, choices, and goals that are theirs alone. We need to be attuned to interpreting non-verbal cues. If the older adult needs help in communicating these cues to the staff (and possibly family members), our commitment to support self-determination requires us to offer that assistance, which might involve providing an advocate to speak for him or her or choosing a time of day when the resident is most capable of participating.

Critical information that can guide decision-making is available from a number of sources. The importance of having accurate and full information about the issue(s) to be decided cannot be overstated, and the decision-maker(s) need to marshal all available factual information that is relevant to consideration of the dilemma. The chart is, of course, an essential source of medical and psychosocial information about a resident. The amount of information that is at hand when a decision needs to be made may vary. Sometimes a care decision needs to be "in the moment," based upon the facts that are at hand or that can quickly be discovered from the chart or other professionals on the floor. At other times, a decision is best made in the context of a care plan meeting or an ethics committee meeting. In these circumstances, available information might include the results of consultations with a psychologist or psychiatrist to determine the care recipient's decisional capacity, a speech therapist to assess the resident's ability to swallow and take nutrition orally, a physical therapist to assess the resident's physical functioning and mobility, and a dietitian to determine how to best meet the resident's nutritional needs. Each of these specialists, as well as others, may participate in the discussion and the decision-making process as appropriate. Finally, family members, too, may be able to provide relevant background and understanding of the resident's history, preferences, and values.

Though full knowledge of the information in a resident's chart and expert evaluations are necessary, they are not sufficient as sources of information about the resident. Knowledge of the elder's *story* as he or she understands and shares it is also essential. Such a personal narrative might be collected and composed piece by piece over time by staff. What we know or do not know of someone else's life story colors our expectations, feelings, judgments, and understanding of that person. Would a particular care decision support that person's self-identity or threaten and perhaps even undermine it?

Step 3: Explore All Potential Options

Step 3 calls for creative thinking by those involved in the decision-making process; it is the "brainstorming" step. The goal of this step is to think of all the possible options for addressing the resident's problem. We are not yet at the point of resolving the ethical dilemma; rather, at this step the object is to be as nonjudgmental and creative as possible in responding to the resident's situation. To encourage new and inventive approaches—anything that responds to the issues raised by the situation— is an appropriate suggestion at this stage. Even suggestions that in themselves would not pass "ethical muster," that violate one or more commitments to the resident, might lead to truly innovative ways to address an ethical dilemma. It is not an easy task to allow ourselves to think outside the box in this way. We automatically judge, censor, assess, and evaluate our own ideas; allowing them free rein is a challenge. However, there can be comfort in the knowledge that evaluation of the suggested responses takes place in Step 4. So with that assurance, allow your creative thinking to flow freely.

Step 4: Assess Each Option

If Step 3 was the "creative thinking" step of the *IDEAS* process, Step 4 is its "critical thinking" step. Participants in the decision-making process evaluate the array of possible responses developed in Step 3. In considering each option, process participants should consider 1) whether it violates any of the commitments long-term care providers have to the receivers of their care; 2) how well it contributes to meeting the commitments to the resident and whether it reflects organizational values; and 3) how well it can be integrated into a plan of care or course of action. Though the five commitments offer a framework for assessing how well the generated care options meet the ethical obligations of long-term care providers, good ethical decisions ultimately depend upon the good judgment and goodwill of the decision-maker(s). How the various possible responses are ultimately weighed and evaluated lies with those charged with the care decision.

Step 5: Select a Course of Action

Rarely does the best solution to a care dilemma in long-term care consist of a single act. The *IDEAS* process encourages the exploration of as wide an array of potential responses to the dilemma as possible, from which a comprehensive course of action can be developed. In Step 5 we identify the what, when, and who of an action plan. We 1) identify the action steps to be taken; 2) determine who will have responsibility for each action step; 3) establish when the action step should be done; and 4) determine how progress will be reported.

In Step 1 of the *IDEAS* process, we identified those persons in addition to the resident who had a stake in the outcome of the process, including family members, staff, and other residents. The ethical dilemma was addressed in light of our commitments to the resident. Nonetheless, to most fully resolve the issue giving rise to our ethical dilemma, an action plan should also include steps that address the concerns of other stakeholders whose interests are affected by the course of action. Such steps might include education of staff and family, grief counseling, efforts at alternative dispute resolution such as mediation, creative ways of including family members in the plan of care, and so forth.

Follow-up to evaluate how well the course of action actually addresses the issue can be very valuable. A record that respects the confidentiality of the client or resident (and complies with relevant provisions of HIPPA) should be kept of the original issue, the decisions that were made, the course of action that was implemented, and the evaluation of the results. Over time, these records will develop as a resource to guide future ethical problem-solving.

IDEAS for Ethical Decision-Making in Long-Term Care

- Identify the ethical dilemma and the stakeholders
- Develop the resident narrative
- Explore all potential options
- Assess each option
- Select a course of action.

Applying *IDEAS* for Ethical Decision-Making

The following illustrates how the *IDEAS* process can be used to resolve the ethical dilemma presented in the case study of Mrs. Hanson set out at the beginning of this chapter.

Step 1: Identify the Ethical Dilemma and the Stakeholders

The first task in approaching this case is to identify the ethical dilemma, that is, to determine which of our ethical commitments to Mrs. Hanson are placed in tension by the situation we are addressing. With the facts as they are reported in the case, a conflict exists between our commitment to preserve and promote Mrs. Hanson's health and our commitments to ease her suffering and pain and continue and complete her life narrative. For those on the team who believe that her resistance to getting on the gurney and to the placement of the arteriovenous catheters is an expression of a choice that she is making to refuse further dialysis, our commitment to preserve her health by continuing dialysis is also in tension with our commitment to respect and support her self-determination. Even at this step, we might need a discussion to clarify which of Mrs. Hanson's interests are at stake.

Stakeholders in this case include Mrs. Hanson, her daughter, the nursing home administrator, the director of nursing, the social worker, staff involved in the care of Mrs. Hanson, and other staff who hold strong beliefs about whether Mrs. Hanson's dialysis should continue. The forum for decision-making might vary from place to place, but all organizations should have an established organizational procedure for addressing ethical dilemmas when they arise. Some organizations might establish an ethics committee to consider ethical issues. Although ethics committees are not as common in nursing home settings as they are in hospitals, an advantage to having an established ethics committee is that the members develop a strong knowledge base and skill in addressing ethical concerns. Alternatively, ethical issues might be addressed at care plan meetings or staff meetings. In general, addressing issues that raise ethical concerns for providers might be more effectively addressed in care plan meetings after the provider(s) have gotten clarity regarding the approach that most fully meets their commitments to the care recipient.

Step 2: Develop the Relevant Information and the Resident Narrative

Here we gather as much information as we can to understand the person who rests at the center of the dilemma. Does Mrs. Hanson have the capacity to provide or withhold informed consent to the continuation of dialysis? If capacity is lacking, has Mrs. Hanson formally designated someone to make decisions for her under the circumstances? The answers to these two questions have legal implications that we need to be aware of. In this case, the answer to both questions is "No." Therefore, we look further, starting with the information in Mrs. Hanson's chart. What is her current health status? What is the most likely course her condition will follow?

Beyond the medical facts, we also want to take account of who Mrs. Hanson is and has been. Given that she is no longer able to verbalize her wishes, we need our familiarity with Mrs. Hanson. Our awareness of her preferences and values, which have been revealed over the years we have known her, allows us to speak on her behalf. Her daughter is another source of information about Mrs. Hanson's life. We can ask her daughter to talk more about the kind of "fighter" her mother was. The purpose of Step 2 is to assure that we are making a decision about the right thing to do for Mrs. Hanson. Rather than basing decisions about medical treatment options upon medical diagnoses, laboratory reports, test results, and prognoses, long-term care affords practitioners, in most cases, the opportunity to develop a much richer narrative of the resident than the facts and data recorded in the chart can provide. "Knowing" someone's life story is more than merely being able to provide descriptive words about her or him. Fulfilling this commitment takes special skill in listening, recognizing important themes, following up with questions, and interpretive understanding of responses. It also takes time and most effectively occurs over time. It is, or can be for those who value this deeper understanding of those for whom they care, a uniquely rewarding opportunity.

Step 3: Explore All Potential Options

One of the advantages of team decision-making is the creative energy that is spurred as members of the team build upon the suggestions offered by colleagues. This step demands uncritical brainstorming. Assessment of the options comes in the next step, so for now suspend judgment and encourage creativity. In the case of Mrs. Hanson, for example, options on the table might include the following:

- Keep taking her out to dialysis, despite her resistance to being put on the gurney and to the catheters
- Give her medication to quiet her on the days when dialysis is scheduled
- Tie Mrs. Hanson down so she can't effectively resist
- Just stop sending Mrs. Hanson for dialysis
- See if her daughter's a match for a kidney transplant
- Ask the chaplain or social worker to speak with Mrs. Hanson's daughter to explore her insistence on continuing dialysis
- See if Mrs. Hanson can be encouraged to give an indication of her wishes (that is, through approaching her at a good time of day, by a social worker, etc.)
- Encourage Mrs. Hanson's daughter to speak with her about her wishes
- Educate Mrs. Hanson's daughter about the physiology of renal dialysis; what is involved for her mother
- Encourage Mrs. Hanson's daughter to go to dialysis with her mother to see for herself what is involved
- See if an exception will be made to allow Mrs. Hanson's daughter to stay with Mrs. Hanson during dialysis
- Check the possibility of receiving dialysis at Green Bower
- Continue dialysis for a limited time with an agreed-upon stop date
- Provide opportunity for listening to staff discuss their feelings and beliefs
- Provide hospice care

Perhaps you might think of other options that are not included in the list.

Step 4: Assess Each Potential Option

The critical faculties are brought into the decision-making process in this step. How does each potential option support our commitments to this recipient of our care? Do any of the suggested options violate our commitments? The assessment of Step 4 includes a legal assessment as well as the ethical assessment. We take note of whether any of the items on the generated list of possible steps is legally required or legally prohibited. Remembering that "ought implies can," we also consider whether any proposed options are simply not possible. If impossible or prohibited options are among the suggestions, they may be removed from among the possible action steps. Occasionally, stakeholders, including the care provider organization itself, may believe so strongly that a particular choice is ethically required that they are willing to assume the legal consequences of acting on that choice, even if it is contrary to existing applicable law.

In this case, among the options generated, "Tie Mrs. Hanson down so she can't effectively resist" is discarded as something we must not do, because it is abusive and contrary to existing laws and regulations regarding restraints. We also need to consider what the law might require us to do. If Mrs. Hanson had executed a living will or health care power of attorney, we generally would be legally obligated to comply with the choices expressed in the living will document or with the decisions made by the person or persons given power of attorney for health care.

We now return to the dilemma we identified in Step 1 to see how the remaining options can help us to reach a resolution, and we begin by reviewing the facts of the case in light of the professional commitments care providers bear toward Mrs. Hanson. The ethical dilemma in this case appears to present a tension between care providers' commitment to Mrs. Hanson's health (that is, the continuation of dialysis, the commitment focused on by staff distressed by the prospect of ending dialysis) and the commitment to relieve her suffering and pain (the focus of staff supporting the decision to stop dialysis). Also implicated are the commitments to respect Mrs. Hanson's self-determination, for which no definitive indication exists, and the continuation of her life story, which her daughter believes supports continued life-sustaining treatment.

Mrs. Hanson never completed an advance directive, nor was she able to discuss her choices regarding medical treatment since her admission to the nursing home. Under the facts we have, her daughter's belief that discontinuing dialysis would be wrong is founded on who she believes her mother to have been (and who she believes her mother continues to be), rather than on any expression by Mrs. Hanson, verbal or nonverbal. Indeed, to the extent that Mrs. Hanson's actions can be understood to express a choice, she appears to be choosing *not* to receive the dialysis.

Her daughter's understanding of the sort of person Mrs. Hanson is and her belief concerning what choices are consistent with Mrs. Hanson's nature and history are very relevant, but they are not reflections of Mrs. Hanson's self-determination. Rather, they are an aspect of her life story and can be considered as the commitment to support that life story is explored in the decision-making process. In this case, we do not have reliable information from Mrs. Hanson herself, expressed verbally or nonverbally, currently or in the past, about what she would choose for herself in this situation, were she able to express a choice.

Without an explicit expression of her self-determination, we turn to exploring Mrs. Hanson's life story to discern what choice would be consistent with that story, so that we can preserve as much as possible its integrity. Mrs. Hanson's daughter's understanding of the person Mrs. Hanson has been is of much relevance. Staff also might have information about how Mrs. Hanson's story has continued since her admission to Green Bower. Has there been a shift in the narrative? Has there been a turn in the story that points in a new direction? Staff might be able to shed light on the most recent chapters of Mrs. Hanson's life story. The commitment here is to continue the life story in a way that does not do violence to it, but rather is faithful to the story created by Mrs. Hanson through the life she actually has lived.

Next, we consider whether continuing dialysis fulfills a commitment to preserve and promote Mrs. Hanson's health. Because most older adults who require long-term care suffer with multiple chronic conditions, the obligation to preserve and promote a resident's health is more often focused on maximizing his or her functional status and ability to participate in his or her own life than it is on curing disease. Sometimes the aggressive treatment, whether medical, surgical, or pharmacological, does not serve the goal of maximizing the ability to engage in those activities that hold value for the resident. In this case, Mrs. Hanson, an 83-year-old woman previously diagnosed with diabetes, osteoarthritis, and dementia, has now developed chronic kidney failure. The continuation of dialysis cannot be expected to lead to generally improved functional status, nor in Mrs. Hanson's ability to participate more fully in her own life. In fact, Mrs. Hanson's health course is on track toward increasing debilitation.

We turn now to consider the fourth commitment implicated in this ethical dilemma—the commitment to ease Mrs. Hanson's suffering and pain. We have reason to interpret her resistance to being taken from her bed and placed on a gurney and then having catheters inserted as being a reaction to pain or discomfort.

Our task at this point is to evaluate the options we generated in Step 3 in light of how we can best fulfill our commitments to Mrs. Hanson. No algorithm exists for carrying out this part of the process. Much thought and discussion is needed. Rarely is the best solution to an ethical dilemma in long-term care a single-step response. Consider all the options and how some or all of them might be combined to resolve the dilemma. One possible assessment: We can't know what Mrs. Hanson would choose for herself under these circumstances. Her life story, as it was explored further with her daughter and staff who came to know her, suggests that, as her daughter said, Mrs. Hanson had been "a fighter." Her daughter was invited to explore this further. As she talked about her mother, she came to realize that for her mother, being able to take care of herself, to have control of events rather than be a passive participant, was very important. She was a fighter because she did not sit on the sidelines of life. Being passive was simply not in her character. Nursing staff proposed providing more information to Mrs. Hanson's daughter about dialysis, what it is, and the prognosis for her mother if she continued with dialysis. The role of hospice care was explained to Mrs. Hanson's daughter. She was assured that her mother would not be abandoned by staff, but would continue to be cared for and to receive whatever she needed to remain comfortable for as long as she lived.

Step 5: Select a Course of Action

This is the step where we develop an action plan. The following is one possible plan:

1. Discuss with Mrs. Hanson's daughter what it meant for her mother to be a fighter; discuss the ways that staff have noticed recently her shift from participation to quiet withdrawal from the activities around her and the significance of these shifts in the dying process.

2. Educate Mrs. Hanson's daughter about the reasons for and limits of dialysis, the role of and services provided by hospice, and what she might expect after dialysis is stopped.

3. Ask the chaplain or social worker to speak with Mrs. Hanson's daughter to address her impending loss.

4. If Mrs. Hanson's daughter agrees, have an order entered in her chart that Mrs. Hanson is not to go out for dialysis.

5. Engage hospice.

6. If and when staff questions the decision, the full process that led to the decision to end dialysis can be shared with them, so that they understand how the decision was reached and that it was not easily, lightly, or capriciously made.

Staff members might be given the opportunity to express their feelings with a social worker or other skilled discussion facilitator.

The suggested course of action is but one possibility for resolving the ethical dilemma posed by the tension among the commitments of long-term care providers to the long-term care recipient in this case. The options offered contain several alternative potential courses of action. How the options are put together in a course of action depends upon the judgment and experience of the individuals engaged in the decision-making process.

Some stakeholders might for various reasons, including religious beliefs, still disagree with the decision to discontinue dialysis for Mrs. Hanson. It might be helpful in those situations to identify an internal mediator, that is, someone who has the trust of the stakeholders and skill in facilitating emotionally charged discussions. Often this can be a social worker or chaplain. If no internal mediator is available, bringing in someone from the outside, either a professional mediator or even someone from a sister long-term care facility that is perceived to be trustworthy might be helpful.

This case illustrates the benefits of implementing a process for resolving ethical dilemmas in long-term care organizations:

1. It provides a process for making team (as opposed to individual) ethical decisions.

2. It establishes a basis for explaining to others how decisions were reached.

3. It permits consistency, reliability, and predictability in the process of ethical decision-making.

4. It provides guidance for addressing unfamiliar or challenging care issues and dilemmas.

5. It counterbalances pressures to make the most expedient decision.

Staff might weigh options differently, and action plans might differ at other times and places. The constant is the commitments long-term care providers make to residents and the process for working through dilemmas when they arise; that is, when those commitments pull toward different choices for a care receiver. Long-term care organizations should keep a record of the outcome of the decisions made and the reasoning behind them, so they become part of the institutional memory. Following up to determine how effective the course of action decided upon is can help guide decision-making in similar situations in the future.

Conclusion

This chapter has described the significant ways in which the provision of long-term care differs from acute care. It has proposed a commitment-based ethical framework that responds to the particular responsibilities and commitments of long-term care providers, as well as a process for resolving ethical dilemmas arising when commitments conflict. Though professionals who practice in long-term care settings have particular areas of expertise, all share a commitment to the well-being of the whole person. The hope is that the ethical approach described in this chapter supports long-term care practitioners in fulfilling that mandate.

Talk About It!

- Think of the definition of an "ethical dilemma." What are several situations you commonly encounter in your work that create tension among your commitments to those for whom you provide care? How do you try to resolve that tension?

- In what ways is the concept of self-determination broader than the concept of autonomy? How might efforts to support self-determination go beyond respecting autonomy?

- What are several of the principal ways in which nursing's role in long-term care differs from that in acute care? Do you find these differences professionally and personally appealing? Why or why not?

References

Beauchamp, T. L., & Childress, J. F. (2008). *Principles of biomedical ethics* (6th ed.). New York, NY:Oxford University Press.

Mathes, M. M., & Menio, D. A. (2007). *Competence with compassion: Ethical decision-making in long-term services and supports.* Philadelphia:Center for Advocacy for the Rights and Interests of the Elderly.

Rachels, J. (1986). *The end of life: Euthanasia and morality.* New York,NY: Oxford University Press.

Self-determination. (n.d.). In the American Heritage Dictionary of the English Language. Retrieved from: http://ahdictionary.com/word/search.html?q=self-determination&submit.x=55&submit.y=28

Walker, M. U. (2007). *Moral understandings: A feminist study in ethics* (2nd ed.) New York, NY: Oxford University Press.

ETHICAL CHALLENGES IN TRANSITIONING TO END-OF-LIFE CARE: EXPLORING THE MEANING OF A "GOOD DEATH"

10

–Gwenyth R. Wallen, PhD, RN
*Chief of Nursing Research and Translational Science,
National Institutes of Health Clinical Center*

–Karen Baker, MSN, CRNP
Pain and Palliative Care Service, National Institutes of Health Clinical Center

Think About It!

- When caring for a patient at the end of life, a nurse must examine her or his own ethical perspectives and the meaning of a "good death," as well as those of the patient and her or his family.

- Advance directives must be verified to examine patient preferences. Printing a copy of the advance directive from the electronic medical record and having it available in the direct care setting are optimal.

- Ongoing assessment of symptom control is paramount and should include exploring unmet psychosocial and spiritual needs.

- When palliative sedation is being considered, assess whether all symptom relieving agents have been maximized.

- Patient care conferences that include the interdisciplinary team, patient, and family should occur early and often.

Nurses are increasingly more aware of the ethical aspects of their practice and how vital these aspects are to the nursing care they provide (Dierckx de Casterlé, Grypdonck, Cannaerts, & Steeman, 2004). Because death is a universal phenomenon, making the end-of-life experience "one of comfort and exquisite care" should be the goal for all nurses (Robley, 2008). This goal is not easy in high-technology health care environments that focus on curing diseases. Few things cause nurses more angst or moral distress than wondering whether they have provided their patients with comfort and dignity at the end of life. Literature has often described this as searching for or providing a "good death."

The first modern hospice geared toward meeting the unmet needs of terminally ill patients and their families was founded in the United Kingdom in 1967 by Dr. Cicely Saunders. At the beginning of the hospice movement, focus was placed on the final days or weeks of a patient's life. In the past few decades, the scope of palliative care has expanded to include earlier stages in the trajectory of incurable diseases (Kaasa & De Conno, 2001; Wallen, Berger, Wittink, & Carr, 2008). The distinct nature and centrality of nurses' roles in the provision of palliative care demand a unique understanding of the potential ethical constraints at the end of life. Nurses will experience value conflicts and challenges to their personal and professional beliefs regarding the meaning of a good death, and at times they will find themselves providing or with-drawing care in a way they find morally objectionable (Scanlon, 1998).

Patients at the end of life present with additional vulnerabilities that require nurses to examine their own ethical perspectives as well as those of the patient and his or her family. Family members often find the provision of end-of-life care to be stressful and burdensome. Experts in the palliative care discipline have sought to inform caregivers who care for individuals at the end of life that death should be meaningful. When possible, a sense of coherence and order must be sought. And the process of dying should make sense not only to the individual and his or her loved ones, but also to the nurses caring for them (Abma, 2005).

What Is Palliative Care, and Where Do Nurses Fit In?

Palliative care is an interdisciplinary, collaborative, individual-centered approach focused on physical, psychosocial, and spiritual care in progressive disease. It focuses both on the quality of life remaining to patients and on supporting their families and those close to them (Higginson, 1999; Wallen et al., 2008). Alleviation from suffering goes beyond physical suffering and includes what is often described as existential suffering. Existential suffering is not well-defined, but generally it is a loss or interruption of meaning, purpose, or hope in life. Existential suffering might also include fear and regret for patients who are knowingly approaching the end of life (Kirk & Mahon, 2010). Patients with advanced malignancies and incurable diseases require customized complements of palliative care, where the emphasis extends beyond pain and symptom management to include the resolution of emotional, social, psychological, and spiritual problems; the provision of information; improved communication; and support for the family (Higginson et al., 2002; Wallen et al., 2008). To be ethical, palliative care should focus on respect for patient autonomy, open awareness, holism, mutual respect, and collaboration among the individual, his or her family and friends, and the health care team (Karim, 2000; Wallen, Ulrich, & Grady, 2005). A study of 91 nurses attending an ethics conference found nurses' main priority centered around their patients' quality of life, which included the obligation to address distressing symptoms, pain, and suffering (Pavlish, Brown-Saltzman, Hersh, Shirk, & Rounkle, 2011). These nurses questioned the benefits and burdens of aggressive medical treatment, particularly at end of life. One respondent—in describing the aggressive treatment of an elderly patient with multiple chronic conditions and poor functional status—questioned whether society can "afford to offer all care to all people" and further noted that "care itself is not without consequences and is often painful." Another respondent described treating an elderly woman with cardiac failure at the end of life and expressed regrets for implementing treatments that caused her more suffering than good: "The health care team was not able to treat the patient appropriately because the family insisted on interventions that could not meaningfully benefit the patient and instead cause discomfort" (Pavlish, et al., 2011, p. 4). Nurses in the study identified 12 ethics-specific nurse activities. The five most frequently identified of the 12 activities included the following:

- Communicating with the health care team in a timely and open manner

- Raising issues promptly and speaking up

- Advocating in the patient's best interest

- Collaborating with families

- Exploring patients' preferences for treatment (Pavlish et al., 2011)

Nurses serve as patient and family advocates with a charge to maintain human dignity and the promise of a good death (Emanuel & Emanuel, 1998). Nurses' compassion for their patients is often the only thing that allows patients to recover or maintain dignity. However, in a hospital setting, a nurse's focus might tend toward basic dignity rather than personal dignity, especially if the nurse lacks the knowledge or understanding of her or his patient as a previously "whole person" (Leung, 2007). For the nurse, the idea of preserving basic dignity might initially focus on meeting physiologic needs, yet the emotional and spiritual needs of the patient might provide a much clearer window into understanding her or his suffering and working toward addressing it in a holistic way. Attention to patients' spirituality in their plan of care is considered to be an ethical and moral obligation for nurses by large professional organizations such as the Canadian Nurses Association (Pesut, 2009).

Over the years, professional discourse and the popular media have brought ethical issues related to care of the dying to the forefront, including the famous cases of Karen Ann Quinlan and Terri Schiavo—both of which have provided frameworks for clinical decision-making at the end of life (Mahon, 2010). Through case studies and vignettes, this chapter examines some of the most common and important clinical questions and ethical issues that confront nurses as they care for their patients at the end of life.

- Can the ethical principles of autonomy be maintained at the end of life?
- Is there a difference between assisted suicide and euthanasia?
- Is it ever appropriate to withdraw hydration or nutrition at the end of life?
- Is palliative sedation ethical?
- How can suboptimal palliative care be addressed?
- What if the goals of care are unclear?

Can the Ethical Principle of Autonomy Be Maintained at the End of Life?

Despite the fact that controversies in decision-making and care are commonplace at the end of life, their potential for exacerbating distress is no less diminished (Scanlon, 1998). Autonomy and self-determination are the ethical and legal terms often used to describe patients' interests at the end of life. Respect for autonomy can lead nurses to processes that preserve their patient as the decision-maker, yet patients might be too ill or choose not to participate in decision-making (Mahon, 2010). When this occurs, nurses might need to partner with physicians and the extended interdisciplinary team to guide patients and their families through a process that elicits their preferences. Subtle but important differences exist between autonomy with a sense of control and the capacity to measure the limits of suffering as opposed to defining life's meaning in suffering (Leung, 2007).

Case Study 10.1

Mrs. H is a 67-year-old metastatic ovarian cancer patient. Her family has asked that she be admitted to the hospital, because she seems lethargic and has seemed confused off and on for the past 24 hours. During her admission assessment on the oncology unit, she seems agitated and is not able to provide the staff with answers to many of the assessment questions that would normally be used to guide her care. Her husband and daughter are present, but when asked to assist in setting goals for her care they seem distraught and state, "Whatever you can do to stop her suffering, do it."

One way of preserving self-determination is through the use of advance directives. The Patient Self-Determination Act, a federal law that went into effect in 1991, requires health care institutions that receive Medicare and Medicaid funding to ask patients whether they have an advance directive. Advance directives are recognized by all states as having legal authority and represent individualized goals of care at the end of life (Meisel, 2008). Living wills represent one type of advance directive and provide guidance to health care providers and families on the types of medical interventions requested if an individual becomes terminally ill. For example, the document can range in specificity and include information on cardiopulmonary resuscitation, analgesia, artificial nutrition and hydration, and antibiotics, among other issues. A durable power of attorney is an advance directive that designates a proxy to make decisions on behalf of an incapacitated adult.

Nurses might be faced with questioning whether the care they are providing is futile. Questions such as these might require them to examine their own views regarding the need for medical treatments that preserve or override their patient's autonomy. The most controversial reason for overriding a patient's autonomy is when the care team reallocates scarce medical resources from a dying patient to promote what might be considered a health systems or organizational decision regarding a more efficient use of resources. There may also be instances when medical care is futile regardless of cost, such as in patients with multi-organ failure at the end of life. This argument might present the withholding of futile care as "ethically obligatory," because care that provides little or no benefit to a dying patient has costs that are "borne in large part by society: by taxpayers through Medicare, Medicaid, or other government programs or through private insurance" (Meisel, 2008, p. 53).

Is There a Difference Between Assisted Suicide and Euthanasia?

In exploring the differences and meanings of assisted suicide and euthanasia, the ethical principle of nonmaleficence—"First, do no harm"—must be taken into account. Clarifying these terms is important both legally and ethically. Physician-assisted suicide is the deliberate action taken by a physician to help a patient commit suicide. In this case, the patient chooses to end his or her life, but the physician provides the means to assist the patient to do so. In the United States, only three states have this statute: Oregon, Washington, and Montana (Kirk & Mahon, 2010). On the other hand, euthanasia is the act of intentionally ending a patient's life and is personally carried out by the health care provider. This is not legal in the United States. U.S. courts have supported rights to refuse care and withdraw care, but not to hasten death.

Case Study 10.2

A.F. is a 30-year-old woman with an end stage immunodeficiency syndrome who has been hospitalized for several months. She has felt as though she has lost control of many things in her life, including her independence, job, and close relationships. She feels completely isolated. Earlier on, she had been discovered to be withholding her own antibiotics therapy. Even with counseling, she is asking, "Why bother? Let me just sleep and not wake up."

The Hospice and Palliative Nurses Association, the National Hospice and Palliative Care Organization, and the Hospice Association of America serve as the United States' leading advocates for terminally ill individuals and their families. As such, these professional associations have taken the lead in establishing position statements to assist in guiding how health care providers should approach the issue of assisted suicides. These positions are evident in statements such as the one addressing the Supreme Court ruling on physician-assisted suicide. Since the 1990s, these groups have supported the premise that laws should not focus on whether the state has an interest in allowing people to ask their physician to help them commit suicide, but rather express that the state has an interest in helping individuals live out their last days as comfortably and dignified as possible. The tenet widely held by these advocates is that when terminally ill patients are given optimal team-oriented medical, nursing, and supportive care for easing symptom burden, the desire for assistance with suicide decreases. The hospice philosophy of care accepts death as a natural part of life and addresses the physiologic, psychosocial, and spiritual needs of the patient and family (http://www.hospicecare.com/Ethics/statements.htm#AAHPM).

Hospice and Palliative Nurses Association's Statement in Response to Supreme Court Ruling on Physician-Assisted Suicide

Hospice and Palliative Nurses Association, Position on Physician-Assisted Suicide, Adopted May 1994. The Hospice and Palliative Nurses Association, the organization that speaks nationally for hospice nurses committed to compassionate care of the terminally ill, having witnessed firsthand the phenomena of palliation, or relief of pain and suffering, and the maintenance of patient/family-defined quality of life of dying patients and their families in hospice care, opposes the legalization of euthanasia and assisted suicide. We reaffirm the hospice concept of care that neither hastens nor postpones the onset of death. In addition, we support all activity toward open discussion, public or private, about these or any other issues that concern hospice patients and families. Finally, we support all public policy changes that would ensure access to hospice care, irrespective of patient age or diagnosis and patient/family socioeconomic status.

http://www.hospicecare.com/Ethics/statements.htm#AAHPM

Is Withdrawing Hydration or Nutrition at the End of Life Ethical?

Limiting hydration or nutrition at the end of life is among the most difficult aspects of care that patients' families and the nurses who care for them face. After all, one might ask how limiting hydration and nutrition can truly support the tenet of nonmaleficence, or do no harm. In fact, at times, hydrating or providing parenteral nutrition might actually cause more pain and suffering for the patient at the end of life.

> ### Case Study 10.3
>
> J.R. is a 77-year-old male with mesenteric cancer with metastasis to liver, pancreas, and colon. He has undergone an extensive surgical Whipple procedure (also know as a pancreaticoduo-denectomy), chemotherapy, and radiation. His jejunostomy feeding tube is not functioning because of the progressive disease and bowel obstruction caused by the growing metastatic tumors. He presents with cachexia, nausea, and abdominal pain. His lungs, liver, and kidneys are beginning to fail. The increased fluids and nutrition are causing edema and increased abdominal and lower extremity pain. His wife wants him to be fed and believes that any reduction in hydration or nutrition is only hastening his death.

In the *New Yorker* essay "Letting Go," Atul Gawande (2010) exemplifies this struggle through the case of Dave Galloway, a 42–year-old firefighter, husband, and father with pancreatic cancer.

> *"The hardest part so far," Sharon (his wife) said, "was deciding to forgo the two-litre intravenous feedings that Dave had been receiving each day. Although they were his only source of calories, the hospice staff encouraged discontinuing them because his body did not seem to be absorbing the nutrition. The infusion of sugars, proteins, and fats made the painful swelling of his skin and his shortness of breath worse—and for what? The mantra was live for now." Sharon balked for fear that she'd be starving him. The night before our visit, however, she and Dave decided to try going without the infusion. By morning, the swelling was markedly reduced. He could move more, and with less discomfort. He also began to eat a few morsels of food, just for the taste of it, and that made Sharon feel better about the decision.*

The issue of initiating artificial hydration and/or nutrition follows physiologic parameters and clinical practice guidelines. The effects these interventions have on overall discomfort, quality of life, appetite loss, and cachexia must also be taken into account. Currently, no conclusive evidence of harm versus benefit of dehydration at the end of life exists.

There are several caregiving tips that nurses can follow when changes in nutrition and hydration are required for optimal care and comfort:

- Recognize the signs of dehydration.

- Role-model other caregiving techniques families can do if they cannot feed the patient, such as gentle touch.

- Appreciate the social, religious, and cultural implication of food for the patient and his or her family and also examine their own values regarding food and mealtime.

Is Palliative Sedation Ethical?

A combination of symptoms causing distress and intractable suffering at the end of life might include delirium, difficulty breathing, pain, nausea, vomiting, myoclonus, anxiety, and depression. These symptoms can often be controlled or at least reduced through the use of pharmacotherapies (Ghafoor & Silus, 2011). Palliative sedation, according to the National Hospice and Palliative Care Organization (NHPCO), is "lowering patient consciousness using medications for the express purpose of limiting patient awareness of suffering that is intractable or intolerable" (Kirk & Mahon, 2010). This is offered to patients who are terminally ill and whose death is imminent. Patients must be unresponsive to other interventions that are less "suppressive of consciousness" (that is, ideally restful but arousable) and suffer from intolerable symptoms. The key factor is the refractory level of the symptom to standard therapies. The level of suffering is measured as unbearable. The pervasive definition of suffering is the "threat to personhood," the unyielding injury, be it physical, psychosocial, spiritual, temporal, or existential in origin.

Case Study 10.4

Mr. J. M., 27, has a history of acute myelodysplastic leukemia requiring a stem cell transplant. He proceeded to have complications from graft versus host disease (GVHD) and infections. The subsequent encephalopathy progressed to a most likely irreversible state. The patient presented with symptoms of moaning, furrowed brow, and rigidity of extremity muscles, with no purposeful movements. Pain medications alone were not effective in decreasing the distressful symptoms that the patient demonstrated. Mr. J. M. was established as a Do Not Resuscitate/Do Not Initiate patient by his durable power of attorney. His family was concerned he was in pain. However, if he was too sleepy, he would not be able to communicate his pain. Sedation was introduced as a mechanism for comfort care measures. The family voiced that they wanted him comfortable, yet they also wanted to interact with him, saying, "If we were to keep him always sedated, would that interrupt a 'miracle'?"

One of the larger studies examining palliative sedation found two primary reasons for initiating sedation: anxiety and confusion/terminal restlessness. Palliative sedation is also implemented for other common symptoms, including dyspnea and refractory pain. The time frame generally used for imminent death is the prognosis of within 14 days. Generally a Do Not Resuscitate order is active, and other intensive interventions, such as dialysis and transfusions, are discontinued. Artificial nutrition/hydration should be discussed with the patient and family prior to initiating sedation. A lack of research exists in this particular area of end of life, so the National Hospice and Palliative Care Organization (NHPCO) encourages health care teams to address the following questions and issues prior to initiating palliative sedation:

- Is palliative sedation an option for the patient?

- Has appropriate proportionality been achieved? Titrate to minimum level of consciousness reduction necessary to render symptoms tolerable.

- Consider interdisciplinary evaluation, including a palliative care physician as lead interventionist, because expertise is required in convening a care conference that is patient- and family-centered.

- Does the facility have ongoing education in palliative sedation competence?

- The bioethical principle of proportionality must be considered where the benefit of the palliative sedation outweighs the burden of that intervention for the individual, where comfort provided by the sedation outweighs the suffering experienced without the sedation.

- Acknowledge that all treatments, including palliative sedation, may have both intended effects as well as unintended adverse consequences, including death. These treatments are considered ethical if they are desirable or helpful to the patient (http://www.eperc.mcw.edu/EPERC).

Nursing actions when caring for a patient receiving palliative sedation should include:

- Reviewing which medications might be decreasing patient awareness.

- Seeking out reasons for progressive underlying distress, including interactions with family and others.

- Assessing whether overall therapy-related side effects might impede coping.

- Pursuing holistic interventions for the patient other than additional medications to decrease symptom burden.

- Gathering a multidisciplinary group in your facility for standards/procedure/policy surrounding the use of palliative sedation.

- Monitoring sedation throughout the process. Knowing how collectively success/efficacy is defined, what parameters do you adjust therapy to?

- Determining who the designated surrogate is for decision-making while the patient is sedated.

As a patient and family advocate, the nurse should continue to coordinate frequent family-care meetings to reconfirm the goals of care. Clear and consistent communication with the family and the care team on how pain in the nonverbal patient is assessed is essential. Family members and friends at the bedside of a loved one who is receiving palliative sedation will often ask the nurse, "How do you know they are not in pain?"

Another important way to keep family members involved is through encouraging them to be at the bedside, to provide comfort care in other ways, and to continue to interact with their loved one. Nurses must continue to serve in an advocacy role for patients and their families as the entire interdisciplinary team works toward providing integrated and "respectful care for people dying with unbearable suffering" (Bruce & Boston, 2010).

What If the Goals of Care Are Unclear? Conflicting End-of-Life Care Goals

The care in the intensive care unit (ICU) traditionally focuses on prolonging survival and curing disease with all that technology has to offer. However, times do exist when families and providers must clarify the goals of care (Mosenthal, 2005). Death should not be seen as a failure and palliative care as a distant second choice to aggressive therapy (Norton & Joos, 2005). Care teams must build a foundation of trust with the patient and their family. Trust that is built on open and ongoing communication can provide the basis for clarifying what the goals of care are.

> ### Case Study 10.5
>
> Mrs. W, 78, underwent surgery for metastatic pancreatic cancer. She has been in the surgical intensive care unit (ICU) for the past 3 weeks on ventilator support because of recurring infection of unknown origin and has experienced multiple bouts of respiratory failure and sepsis. Her family shares that because of her advanced age, she would not want to be maintained on these machines for the rest of her life. The patient had also shared this with her physicians before the surgery. The nurses taking care of Mrs. W feel that the ongoing life support is prolonging her suffering, yet the surgeon's notes state that the prognosis for survival is excellent and that with time, slow ventilator weaning, and improved nutrition, her condition might improve. Therefore, the surgeon's goal for her care is discharge.

Because nurses caring for the patient at the end of life spend long periods of time with the patient and his or her loved ones, they might be the care team member who first discovers a disconnect exists in the goals of care. In the case of Mrs. W, the nurses caring for her need to approach the surgical team, express their concerns, and ask for clarification as to the realistic prognosis the team should expect. The nurses should also confirm care goals with Mrs. W's family after the goals have been clarified with the ICU and surgical teams.

Questions that a nurse might ask patients and their families to guide valuable discussions to validate goals of care at the end of life include the following:

- With your current condition, what is most important for you right now? What are you hoping for? What do you hope to avoid?

- What are you expecting for the time you have left?

- What are you afraid might happen?

- What are your goals for this last phase of your life?

Conclusion

To maximize their therapeutic relationship with the dying patient, nurses must be present for their patients. This sense of presence allows the nurse to fully engage in the care of a dying patient by focusing on comfort and symptom relief, while respecting the patient's and family's psychosocial and spiritual needs.

Striving to work toward providing a "good death" for patients requires nurses to face their own values and potential fears regarding death. Advocacy includes informing and supporting both the dying patient and his or her family. Nurses are not called upon to act in place of the patient, but rather as an advocate. Experience brings strength to the advocacy role for nurses and to end-of-life care. Fear, including fear of the unknown, can become a barrier to advocacy (Thacker, 2008). As advocates, nurses need to exercise ethical assertiveness during interdisciplinary rounds and advocate further for the role of the nurse as an active participant in ethical decisions (Norton & Joos, 2005). With new knowledge and experience surrounding the ethical issues at the end of life come the responsibility and accountability for striving to advocate for a good death that exemplifies a holistic approach to dying. Table 10.1 offers additional web-based resources, so the reader may access further information on many ethical issues addressed in this chapter.

Table 10.1 Resources on Ethical Issues and Palliative Care

Organization Name	Website
The Hastings Center	http://www.thehastingscenter.org/
International Association of Hospice and Palliative Care	http://www.hospicecare.com/Ethics/
American Academy of Hospice and Palliative Medicine	http://www.aahpm.org/
Hospice and Palliative Nurses Association	http://www.hpna.org/
Americans for Better Care of the Dying	http://www.abcd-caring.org
End of Life/Palliative Education Resource Center	http://www.eperc.mcw.edu/EPERC
Companion website for *On Our Own: Moyers on Dying* series	http://www.pbs.org/wnet/onourownterms

Talk About It!

- Have you or your colleagues written out your own advance directives? How comfortable would you feel discussing advance directives with your parents? Siblings? Children? Or friends and those in your community? If nurses cannot bring themselves to do it, how can we expect others to? Consider pushing yourself past your comfort level and beginning conversations about creating advance directives with your colleagues and then continue having the discussions in your family and community groups.

- What can we give the family to do that is tangible at the bedside so they feel like they are providing comfort in lieu of feeding the patient? Discuss options with your colleagues and come up with suggestions to apply as the need arises.

- How does "suffering" manifest in a dying patient? Discuss with your colleagues.

References

Abma, T. (2005). Struggling with the fragility of life: A relational-narrative approach to ethics in palliative nursing. *Nursing Ethics, 12*(4), 337-348.

Bruce, A., & Boston, P. (2011). Relieving existential suffering through palliative sedation: Discussion of an uneasy practice. *Journal of Advanced Nursing* [Epub ahead of print]. doi: 10.1111/j.1365-2648.2011.05711.x

Dierckx de Casterlé, B., Grypdonck, M., Cannaerts, N., & Steeman, E. (2004). Empirical ethics in action: Lessons from two empirical studies in nursing ethics. *Medicine, Health Care and Philosophy, 7*(1), 31-39.

Emanuel, E., & Emanuel, L. (1998). The promise of a good death. *The Lancet, 351*(suppl. II), 21-29.

Gawande, A. (2010, August 2). Letting go. *The New Yorker.*

Ghafoor, V., & Silus, L. S. (2011). Developing policy, standard orders, and quality-assurance monitoring for palliative sedation therapy. *American Journal of Health System Pharmacy, 68*(6), 523-527.

Higginson, I. J. (1999). Evidence based palliative care: There is some evidence—and there needs to be more. *British Medical Journal, 319*(7208), 462-463.

Higginson, I. J., Finlay, I., Goodwin, D. M., Cook, A. M., Hood, K., Edwards, A. G., . . . Norman, C. E. (2002). Do hospital-based palliative teams improve care for patients or families at the end of life? *Journal of Pain Symptom Management, 23*(2), 96-106.

Kaasa, S., & De Conno, F. (2001). Palliative care research. *European Journal of Cancer, 37*(Suppl. 8), S153-S159.

Karim, K. (2000). Conducting research involving palliative patients. *Nursing Standard 15*(2): 34-36.

Kirk, W., Mahon, M., & Palliative Sedation Task Force of the National Hospice and Palliative Care Organization Ethics Committee. (2010). National Hospice and Palliative Care Organization (NHPCO) position statement and commentary on the use of palliative sedation in imminently dying terminally ill patients. *Journal of Pain and Symptom Management, 39*(5), 914-920.

Leung, D. (2007). Granting death with dignity: Patient, family, and professional perspectives. *International Journal of Palliative Nursing, 13*(4), 170-174.

Mahon, M. M. (2010). Clinical decision making in palliative care and end of life care. *Nursing Clinics of North America, 45*(3), 345-362.

Meisel, A. (2008). End-of-life care. In M. Crowley (Ed.), *From birth to death and bench to clinic: The Hastings Center bioethics briefing book for journalists, policymakers, and campaigns* (pp. 51-54). Garrison, NY: The Hastings Center.

Mosenthal, A. C. (2005). Palliative care in the surgical ICU. *Surgical Clinics of North America, 85*(2), 303-313.

Norton, C., & Joos, O. (2005). Caring for Catherine: A cry to support ethical activism. *Journal of Pediatric Oncology, 22*(2), 119-120.

Pavlish, C., Brown-Saltzman, K., Hersh, M., Shirk, M., & Rounkle, A. (2011). Nursing priorities, actions, and regrets for ethical situations in clinical practice. *Journal of Nursing Scholarship, 43*(4), 385-395. DOI: 10.1111/j.1547-5069.2011.01422.x.

Pesut, B. (2009). Incorporating patients' spirituality into care using Gadow's ethical framework. *Nursing Ethics, 16*(4), 418-428.

Robley, L. (2008). From ethics to palliative care: A community hospital experience. *Nursing Clinics of North America, 43*(3), 469-476.

Scanlon, C. (1998). Unraveling ethical issues in palliative care. *Seminars in Oncology Nursing, 14*(2), 137-144.

Thacker, K. (2008). Nurses' advocacy behaviors in end of life nursing care. *Nursing Ethics, 15*(2), 174-185.

Wallen, G. R., Berger, A., Wittink, H., & Carr, D. (2008). Palliative care outcome measures: Translating research into practice. In H. Wittink & D. Carr, *Pain management: Evidence, outcomes, and quality of life, A sourcebook.* Chatswood, NSW: Elsevier.

Wallen, G. R., Ulrich, C., & Grady, C. (2005). Learning about a "good death": Ethical considerations in palliative care nursing research. *DNA Reporter, 30*(2), 8-9.

ETHICAL ISSUES IN NEONATAL NURSING

11

–Elizabeth Gingell Epstein, PhD, RN
Assistant Professor
University of Virginia School of Nursing

Think About It!

- Neonatal nurses encounter ethical issues every day and play an important role in preventing and resolving ethical conflict.

- One of the most pressing ethical concerns today in neonatal ethics is how nurses and other health care providers communicate with each other and with parents.

- Strategies for identifying and acting on common triggers of ethical conflict are provided.

Ethics is an inescapable aspect of neonatal nursing. Consciously or not, neonatal nurses practice ethics in some way on every shift. Balancing benefits and burdens; advocating for infants and parents; maintaining confidentiality; promoting privacy; and speaking carefully and truthfully with colleagues and parents—all require ethical judgment. Most encounters with ethics do not involve conflict. Instead, making judgment calls independently and speaking up for those who cannot speak take center stage. Supporting parents when they need support is also a frequent factor. Simply put, encounters with neonatal ethics situations involve respecting the dignity of human beings.

When ethical conflict does occur, some nurses might feel as though the issues at hand are outside the nursing realm (for example, end-of-life decisions), or that they do not possess the ethics knowledge necessary to participate in a difficult conversation. The nursing role might not include making treatment decisions, but nurses play an important role in helping to resolve ethical conflicts because:

- Nurses are highly familiar with underlying factors, such as ineffective communication, inconsistent providers, or unrealistic expectations that precede the conflict.

- Daily encounters with ethical issues prepare nurses well for participation in ethically challenging situations.

- Nurses have a unique vantage point in that they know their patients well, understand parents' fears and needs, and are knowledgeable about the medical diagnosis and treatment decisions being discussed.

This chapter includes four sections. First, the historical influences on neonatal ethics are briefly reviewed. Second, four infant cases are presented that describe commonly occurring ethical issues in neonatal nursing. Third, important clinical and environmental factors for neonatal ethics are identified. Finally, the neonatal nurse's role in identifying and preventing ethical challenges, including potential strategies for addressing ethical issues in the field, is discussed.

Historical Background of Neonatal Ethics

Several landmark cases from the 1970s and 1980s ignited the field of neonatal ethics. These cases led directly to the enactment of federal laws. Though meant to protect disabled infants, these laws were viewed by many as encroachments on the privacy of the provider-parent relationship and as threats to medical authority. In short, the "Baby Doe" laws, as they are often called, caused a storm in neonatology in the 1980s, and the echoes of that storm continue to ripple through the field today.

Baby Doe was born in Bloomington, Indiana, in 1982 with Down syndrome, esophageal atresia, and tracheoesophageal fistula (Weir, 1984). After much deliberation, the parents, with the support of several physicians, decided against surgical intervention or intravenous hydration, with the understanding that this would lead to the infant's death. This case, and several others occurring around the same time, spurred several difficult ethical questions: "Who decides?" "What are the limits of parental authority?" "What is quality of life?"

The federal government became involved in several cases, including Baby Doe, and instituted the "Baby Doe" rules (Weir, 1984). Under this law, institutions are forbidden to withhold or withdraw treatment (including nutrition, hydration, and medical interventions) from an infant unless the infant is chronically and irreversibly comatose, the provision of treatment would merely prolong dying, or the provision of treatment would be inhumane and futile in terms of the infant's survival (USDHHS, 1985).

The penalty for neglecting to provide treatment was withdrawal of federal funding (which nearly every health care institution relies upon to some degree). Moreover, the delivery rooms, pediatric wards, newborn nurseries, and neonatal intensive care units (NICUs) in these institutions were required to post a placard stating, "Discriminatory failure to feed and care for handicapped infants in this facility is prohibited by federal law. Failure to feed and care for infants may also violate the criminal and civil laws of your state" (Weir, 1984, p. 133). A toll-free number was provided so that anyone—parent, provider, visitor—could report suspected neglect.

Needless to say, this period of time was one of great upheaval in regard to the physician-parent relationship and decision-making for critically ill newborns. Wide debate and great uncertainty about the law's interpretation were the norm (Kopelman, 2005; Kopelman, Irons, & Kopelman, 1988). Further, the demeaning language, fear of litigation, and threat of withdrawal of federal funding have contributed to a "treat until certain" philosophy that still exists in many NICUs throughout the country (Campbell & Fleischman, 2001; Penticuff, 1998).

The questions raised by the Baby Doe case and others of the time continue to arise in neonatal nursing ethics. The range of ethical questions encountered by neonatal nurses has broadened beyond these questions, however. With the advent of increasingly complex technologies come questions about defining the borders of appropriate therapy. With the swing of the pendulum toward parental authority in decision-making come questions about how best to share this sometimes heavy burden. And, with the increasing shift toward a multiprofessional team care approach and the empowerment of nurses comes recognition of the accountability and contribution of nurses to the team and patient.

Four Cases Exhibiting Common Ethical Issues

Case Study 11.1

Baby boy M was born at full term with a congenital heart defect and no other apparent abnormalities. He was admitted to the NICU and immediately required near-maximal life support. Over the next several days, three cardiologists and a cardiac surgeon examined the infant and agreed the defect was irreparable.

A neonatologist and cardiologist met with the parents and described the infant's condition, stating that no treatment would fix his heart and that he could not survive. The parents adamantly refused withdrawal of treatment and insisted that their son be kept alive "no matter what." At one point in a conversation with the parents, a treatment option, extracorporeal membrane oxygenation (ECMO), was offered that would "buy some time" with their son. The parents readily agreed. After 3 weeks of treatment, Baby M's clinical picture had improved significantly. He had become much less edematous, and medications to support his blood pressure were weaned considerably.

However, although he remained sedated, he responded to painful procedures, and even diaper and position changes appeared to cause him some degree of distress, as he grimaced and required increased oxygen and prolonged periods of rest and calming after even the slightest care. The nursing staff was increasingly troubled by his apparent suffering. They and the doctors recognized that Baby M had improved only because the ECMO machine was working more efficiently than his own heart ever would, and that he could not survive off the ECMO machine for long. Baby M's parents, however, saw the dramatic change in their son's physical appearance and knew that his medications were decreasing, and they were filled with hope.

Despite numerous frank discussions, the parents were unbending in their conviction that everything be done. They described themselves as religiously orthodox and were steadfast in their belief that prayer would bring a miracle. During Baby M's hospital stay, there was increasing discontent among the nurses and physicians. Some (both nurses and physicians) were so distraught by his suffering and so angered by the parents' "inability to see reality" they agreed to share the burden by rotating providers frequently. As a result, Baby M and his family rarely saw the same nurse twice in 1 week or had the same physician more than 2 or 3 days in a row.

This case presents a dilemma of balancing beneficence (do no harm) with two aspects of autonomy (doing what is best for Baby M and parental authority in decision-making). This case also raises questions of the appropriateness of prolonged, aggressive treatment, appropriate use of resources (justice), and futility. Additional contextual factors (spirituality and inconsistent providers) influence the way parental authority and Baby M's best interests are balanced. These factors are discussed in the section "Clinical and Environmental Factors Influencing Ethically Challenging Situations" later in the chapter.

Autonomy: Decisional Authority of Parents and the Best Interests Standard

Western society places great value on the principle of autonomy. Parental authority is often viewed as one type of autonomy, as no other relationship (husband/wife, sister/brother, doctor/patient) is quite the same in terms of accountability, responsibility, dependence, or emotional attachment. Health care organizations are reluctant to overstep this authority, so health care providers tend to give wide berth to parents in their decision-making.

However, this authority has its limits. Parents do not have the authority to demand treatments that are overly burdensome (on balance with the benefits to the child) or that would not be acceptable to a reasonable adult (Beauchamp & Childress, 2009). Health care providers are not required to give in to such demands. It seems clear that continued treatment for Baby M is not supported by this aspect of autonomy. Why then does this type of acquiescence occur? To answer this question, nurses need to understand how decisions are contemplated in ethics.

Nurses can use several ethical frameworks to analyze an ethical challenge. First, the four key principles of autonomy, beneficence, nonmaleficence, and justice are frequently called upon in ethical decision-making (Beauchamp & Childress, 2009). These principles help providers to answer difficult questions that develop in neonatal nursing:

- Who can make decisions for a patient (if not the patient himself)?

- What benefits and burdens exist with each possible treatment option?

- How are resources (supplies, beds, staffing, technology, etc.) being used to identify ethically justifiable options for a patient?

However, the principles framework does have shortcomings. It does not always take into account the context (especially the social or environmental contexts) of a particular case, nor does it recognize the importance of maintaining key relationships as an ethical obligation. A different framework, the ethic of care, does take into account context and relationships as central tenets (Carse, 1991; Gilligan, 1987).

The ethic of care framework requires a close look at key relationships involved in the case. In Baby M's case, maintaining the provider-parent relationship and the relationship between parents and baby are ethical obligations. Nurse-parent and doctor-parent relationships are foundational to neonatal nursing and medical practice, because they allow providers to know the parents—their perspectives, fears, and priorities. This is crucial in ensuring good patient care and in supporting parents in decision-making.

For Baby M, withdrawing aggressive treatment without the parents' agreement (or at least their acceptance) would risk destroying not only the provider-parent relationship, but also parents' perceptions of their role as parent (protector and advocate). Unilateral withdrawal of life support would risk leaving parents with empty arms, resentment against health care providers, and a terribly sad picture of their infant's last moments of life. Though the short-term, ethically right action might be to withdraw aggressive treatment for Baby M, the long-term, ethically right action might be to move more slowly toward this end to preserve parents' integrity as parents and human beings. This is one rationale for the acquiescence that is seen in Baby M's case and in other similar cases. However, this perspective does *not* justify continued acquiescence or the use of unrealistic or ineffective therapies. Acknowledging the importance of the provider-parent and parent-child relationships is simply one piece of a complex clinical situation that should be considered in the discussion.

A second aspect of autonomy arises when dealing with situations in which decisions must be made for people (infants) who have never possessed competence—who have never made their desires and wishes known. These situations are different from those involving previously competent people, such as a previously healthy 30-year-old woman who sustains a severe brain injury and is unable to communicate her wishes. In this case, a surrogate decision-maker and health care team would base treatment decisions on what the patient *would have wanted*, whether or not they ever actually or specifically articulated these desires. This avenue for decision-making cannot be followed for neonates. Instead, decisions are made based on what would be in the infant's *best interest* (Beauchamp & Childress, 2009). This standard holds that the surrogate decision-maker should weigh the benefits and harms of the different options and make decisions based on the option that potentially yields the highest benefit, using the rationale of "what a reasonable person would choose" (Beauchamp & Childress, 2009; Weir, 1984). For example, circumstances that render an infant continuously tortured yet alive must be weighed against the nothingness yet ended suffering of death, however painful the act of weighing these two options might be. The harm of continued existence might outweigh the harm of death from a reasonable person perspective. With a uniformly poor prognosis, the best interests standard would support providing Baby M with as peaceful and pain-free a life and death as possible. Again, the best interests standard is simply one piece of a complex puzzle. It is added to the discussion along with the importance of maintaining relationships and the authority of parents to make decisions for their children.

 ## PURPOSE EXERCISE: CONSIDER AND WRITE YOUR ANSWERS TO THE FOLLOWING QUESTIONS

1. Have you encountered a situation in which a parent desired (and authorized) a treatment that you believed was not in the infant's best interest?

2. What evidence was there that the treatment was not in the infant's best interest?

3. What was your role?

4. How did the situation resolve?

5. Did it resolve in a satisfactory way, in your opinion?

6. Why or why not?

Futility

The concept of futility dates back at least to Hippocrates, who instructed his students that they should "refuse to treat those who are overmastered by their disease, realizing that in such cases medicine is powerless" (Chadwick & Mann, 1983). This same idea holds true today—that physicians are not obligated to provide treatment they believe will be ineffective or futile (Council on Ethical and Judicial Affairs, 1999). However, the term *futility* is highly controversial in ethics, largely because defining it is dependent on one's goals or values (Kasman, 2004; Truog, Brett, & Frader, 1992).

- From a *goals perspective*, suppose the goal for Baby M is to improve his circulation. In that case, ECMO worked (and is, therefore, not futile). Baby M's condition (circulation and ventilation) improved dramatically. If the goal is to improve Baby M's chances for survival or to provide a treatment that will allow him to survive, then ECMO is an abysmal failure and could be deemed futile.

- From a *values perspective*, Baby M's parents see great value in continued treatment because it keeps their son alive. Baby M's nurses and doctors, on the other hand, see no value in continued treatment, because the long-term goal of survival cannot be met. Futility is, therefore, not so clear-cut as one might think.

For health care providers, discussing the values and goals that exist and why a treatment might be deemed futile can be helpful in terms of redefining the treatment goals for a patient. For patients and families, using the word *futile* is not likely to be as helpful because of the wide variation in interpretation. Instead, discussing the benefits and burdens of treatment options is more productive in helping families understand a complicated situation (Jonsen, Siegler, & Winslade, 2006).

PURPOSE EXERCISE: CONSIDER AND WRITE YOUR ANSWERS TO THE FOLLOWING QUESTIONS

1. Have you encountered a situation in which you believed the treatment being applied to a patient was "futile"?

2. What was your interpretation of the word?

3. How might your interpretation have been different from another's interpretation?

Suffering and Prolonged Aggressive Treatment

Nurses are keenly aware of patient suffering. Most patients will suffer, at least to some extent, during illness. Nurses can and do attend to this suffering as best they can with the knowledge that, often, all suffering cannot be relieved. Nurses face little ethical difficulty in dealing with short-term suffering when the long-term gains are significant. We do not agonize (ethically) over the patient with postoperative pain after an appendectomy or the premature infant having blood drawn via heel stick. We do, however, agonize deeply and ethically when we inflict suffering, such as suctioning, IV insertions, and heel sticks, on patients for whom the long-term outcome is not good, as is true for Baby M.

Like suffering, prolonged aggressive treatment is sometimes an appropriate expectation. The 27-week gestation premature infant is expected to endure months-long treatment, as is the infant with congenital diaphragmatic hernia. The outcomes for these infants are typically good, making the long duration of treatment worthwhile. Also like suffering, we have a limit to our ability to tolerate the burden of prolonged aggressive treatment for a patient when the outcomes are likely to be poor.

Moral Distress

These situations can lead to moral distress among providers. Moral distress occurs when one believes he or she knows the right action to take (in Baby M's case, it is to withdraw aggressive treatment and promote a peaceful, dignified death), but cannot take that action because of constraints (here, the difficulty is balancing parental authority with the infant's best interests—and for nurses, whose role is not to make treatment decisions, the lack of power). See Epstein & Delgado, 2010, for more in-depth discussion of this topic.

Justice: The "Technological Imperative" and the Use of Scarce Resources

Technological advancements have pushed the field of neonatal ethics. Discoveries including oxygen, intravenous nutrition, cardiorespiratory monitors, surfactant, neonatal resuscitation programs, mechanical ventilation, and ECMO have challenged ethical thinking all along the way. Knowing when to employ these technologies and when to withhold them is not always an easy decision.

Additionally, the historical background has set a precedent that aggressive therapies should be used to comply with the law. As a result, NICUs often support aggressive treatment, using all available treatments until survival of the infant is almost certainly not possible. This philosophy can be viewed as having little regard for infant suffering, engendering false hope, unnecessarily using scarce resources, and driving up health care costs. Alternatively, it can also be viewed as providing opportunities to learn from situations to improve care for future infants and reassuring parents that providers have "tried everything." For decades now, organizations have placed increasing emphasis on employing complex technologies to the point that a "technological imperative"—an impulse to use technologies because they are available, not because they are necessarily in the best interest of the patient—appears to take precedence. As Fuchs stated more than 40 years ago, the only "legitimate and explicitly recognized constraint is the state of the art" (Fuchs, 1968).

The technological imperative is driven by many things, including patient and family expectations, fear of litigation, and a view that the use of technology is a moral or professional responsibility (Hofman, 2002). Fortunately, organizations are increasing their awareness of this phenomenon and more providers are now asking, "Just because we can, should we?" This topic will continue to be a key issue—not only in neonatal practice but in adult critical care as well—especially as health care costs and resources become important factors in decision-making.

Simply put, the principle of justice describes the distribution of goods. How these goods are distributed makes this principle highly complex. Should goods be distributed to those who need them most or those who would benefit from them most? Suppose that Baby M is the only patient on the unit for whom ECMO might be needed. Aside from the question as to Baby M's actual need, if no other patient is on the unit, no obvious resource crisis in employing the therapy exists. Suppose, however, that an infant with persistent pulmonary hypertension (PPHN) is admitted to the unit. Her outcomes would be excellent if she was put on ECMO, but would be very poor if ECMO was not available. Baby M cannot benefit from ECMO in the same way as the new infant. Should Baby M be taken off ECMO to save this new baby, or does the fact that Baby M is currently using the machine give him some claim to that machine?

Goods include not only technologies but personnel, beds, and procedures. Nurses face the question of how goods are distributed daily—when ICU beds are allotted, when nurses are shifted to other units in order to "fill holes" in staffing, when surgical procedures are delayed to allow emergency procedures to be done, and so on.

The role of nurses in cases such as Baby M is not to conduct an ethical analysis or to make treatment decisions. Instead, nurses can help bring ethical conflict to light, providing useful contextual and clinical information. Nurses are not required to recognize the ethical issues at play (such as parental authority, best interests, or use of scarce resources), but such recognition can help shed light on individual influential factors involved in the situation. And acknowledging that a particular clinical situation has stirred angst among the staff; has created a rift among doctors, nurses, or parents; or does not feel right for whatever reason is well within the nurse's purview. That contextual information could include the parents' perspectives, their fears, and the depth of their understanding of the problems their child faces. Nurses are adept at collecting certain types of clinical information, such as subtle changes in personality, physical activity, tone, stool patterns, and feeding tolerance—all of which can add to the objective data (lab results, x-rays, vital signs, medication titrations) to create a full clinical picture.

Case Study 11.2

Baby girl G was a 23-week-gestation, 410-gram infant born following precipitous preterm labor. In the delivery room, she was noted to be blue and floppy but did demonstrate some respiratory effort. The delivery team decided that she should be resuscitated and taken to the NICU for further evaluation. On day of life three, the nurse noted seizure-like activity in her upper limbs, a noticeable decrease in overall tone, and blood pressure instability. A head ultrasound later revealed a severe bilateral intraventricular hemorrhage. The team agreed that a "watch and wait" approach was appropriate as they attempted to stabilize her seizures and blood pressure. Over the next few days, her condition did indeed stabilize. However, her overall tone continued to be very poor. The team met with Baby G's parents to discuss her condition. The parents seemed to understand the issues their infant was having, but they asked that everything be done for her. After this meeting, the parents did not visit their infant for 2 weeks, although the mother did call about every day or two. During this time, the team had increasing trouble with a lack of consensus about how treatment should proceed and whether or not further treatment was necessary. Some argued that Baby G was obviously neurologically devastated and that further aggressive treatment was inhumane. Others argued that telling how infants like Baby G will fare in the future is difficult and that it was too soon to "give up." In the staff lounge one evening, a resident and nurse were discussing Baby G's condition and the resident stated, "I'm not even sure why she was resuscitated in the delivery room. How many 23-weekers survive anyway?" The nurse agreed and said, "Now that she's got all this technology supporting her, it'll be impossible to take that all away and let her go."

In the Baby G situation, the ethical challenge is this: Is it best to withdraw aggressive therapies and allow her to die, or is it best to continue treatment and to help her to survive, because there is some uncertainty as to her long-term neurological status? Further, the resident and nurse question the idea of resuscitation in the delivery room for infants of this gestational age and the apparent difficulty of withdrawing life-sustaining treatment. These issues—prognostic uncertainty, withdrawal versus withholding aggressive treatment, delivery room resuscitation, and quality of life—are key ethical issues present here.

Prognostic Uncertainty

"Currently there is no settled consensus—in fact there is not even the most rudimentary agreement—about what circumstances justify abating aggressive NICU therapies" (Penticuff, 1998). We have generally no way to predict, at birth or even at points during the NICU stay, whether an infant will survive or die, have multiple disabilities, or have none. We can identify some infants as highly unlikely to survive (for example, Baby M or an infant with Trisomy 18) and some infants as highly likely to survive (for example, an otherwise healthy 34-week gestation infant with hyperbilirubinemia). However, for infants who reside in the uncomfortably broad gray area of prognostic uncertainty, the risk/benefit ratio of continued aggressive treatment becomes difficult to calculate. Providers' ability to predict survival and death has been shown to be unreliable in clinical situations where accurate prediction would be helpful (Frick, Uehlinger, & Zuercher Zenklusen, 2003; Meadow et al., 2002). Providers seem able to predict accurately many patients who ultimately survive and many patients who ultimately die. However, a significant and problematic proportion of patients for whom neither survival nor death are predicted accurately remains (Frick et al., 2003; Meadow et al., 2002). Prognostic uncertainty is unsettling for health care providers and parents alike, but is a constant reality in the neonatology and intensive care settings (van Zuuren, & van Manen, 2006).

Withdrawal Versus Withholding

From an ethics standpoint, withdrawing a therapy already started is the same as not starting it in the first place (Beauchamp & Childress, 2009). Weighing and balancing harms and benefits (the principles of beneficence and nonmaleficence) are critical. Beneficence and nonmaleficence address the topic of harm—whether preventing harm, removing harm, or not inflicting harm in the first place. In cases where withdrawal of life-sustaining treatment is in question, caregivers have to ask whether the burdens of continued treatment are harmful when weighed against the burdens of withdrawal. Unfortunately, in some situations death is less burdensome than a life of prolonged agony or in situations where long-term survival is impossible.

Recall here the issues of suffering and futility. A treatment that serves only to keep a brain-dead patient's heart beating gives a caregiving team little reason to continue the therapy. Likewise, not starting a therapy that is believed to have no potential benefit is ethically permissible. Beginning dialysis on an infant born with renal agenesis and hypoplastic lung syndrome is of no benefit, for example. Often, an infant's condition is not fully known prior to delivery, nor does a team know whether or not a treatment will be beneficial. In such instances, a "trial of therapy" is initiated to fully assess the situation. Repeated assessments over time can help define more clearly the benefits and harms. This process has occurred for both Baby M and Baby G.

Baby M's heart condition was so severe that long-term survival was impossible. Thus, starting aggressive treatment would not have helped him, and stopping aggressive treatment would not have harmed him. The problem is, however, that the extent of his cardiac defect was unknown at the time of his birth. Starting aggressive therapies was necessary to properly assess his condition. There was potential, in those early days, for aggressive therapies to be helpful. What if his defect had been surgically reparable? In that case, not starting treatment (withholding) would have certainly been harmful. Baby M would have died unnecessarily. Baby G is in a similar situation.

Suppose that Baby Girl G had been born at 20 weeks' gestation. She would have had no chance for survival, even with all the current technologies available. The burdens of therapy clearly outweigh any potential benefits, and withholding treatment is an ethically appropriate response. However, Baby G was born at 23 weeks gestation, which represents the cusp in terms of survival statistics (Lantos & Meadow, 2006). Neonatologists might opt to resuscitate these infants in the delivery room (a trial of therapy). In the delivery room, the potential for survival exists—the benefits might outweigh the harms. However, the risk of severe handicap is also high. Now, however, Baby G has suffered a serious setback, reducing her chances for long-term survival overall and increasing her risk for survival with severe and debilitating handicaps. Do the benefits of treatment continue to outweigh the harms at this point? This is the ethical question currently being debated in this case.

PURPOSE EXERCISE: CONSIDER AND WRITE YOUR ANSWERS TO THE FOLLOWING QUESTIONS

1. What are your thoughts with regard to withholding and withdrawing life-sustaining treatment?

2. Do you agree with the idea that withholding life-sustaining treatments that will not work is ethically identical to withdrawing life-sustaining treatments that are not working?

Although no ethical difference between withholding and withdrawing ineffective treatments exists, many providers see the emotional differences as substantial. Withdrawing a treatment seems much more difficult than to withhold it altogether, as noted by Baby G's nurse and resident. The well-justified trials of therapy can easily turn into lengthy, complicated, and ethically challenging situations. In such situations, maintaining a focus on patient-centered care can help to steer discussions toward the development of a clearly defined set of treatment goals, thus establishing a base for review and accountability. Establishing a strong nurse-parent relationship early on is useful when complications and complexities arise, as honest and open discussions about harms and benefits as well as understanding parents' viewpoints, fears, and wishes are necessary to decide which treatment path is most appropriate.

Quality of Life

For Baby G, the quality of her life, both now and in the future, is in question. Will she be handicapped? To what degree? What constitutes a "good" quality of life? Recall the case of Baby Doe, who was born with Down syndrome and associated congenital gastrointestinal anomalies. In the 1980s, assuming that surgical repair of his gastrointestinal anomalies would be successful was reasonable. Yet, the parents and physician chose to withhold these surgeries knowing that the baby would die. Presumably, this choice was made as a judgment about the infant's quality of life. This and a variety of other cases in the 1980s shed light on the tenuous nature of quality of life judgments as value-laden and treacherous. Further, recent work has suggested that providers are not accurate in their predictions of patients' quality of life (Frick et al., 2003).

On the other hand, the topic must be broached for some children, and Baby G is a good example. The kind of life she might lead, as uncertain as that is, should be discussed with her parents. Campbell and

McHaffie have argued, "To leave them [quality of life judgments] out is to ignore the practical realities of caring for children with catastrophic impairments and to undervalue the importance of compassion in patient care" (1995, p. 340). Lantos and Meadow (2006) suggest a four-pronged approach to thinking about quality of life: "1) the anticipated cognitive…function, 2) the anticipated physical disabilities, 3) the pain and suffering that is associated with the disease, and 4) the burdens of the treatments that will be necessary in the future" (p. 80). This approach allows for a clearer picture of the underlying problems faced by an individual patient while still leaving plenty of room for insertion of individual values, because how one person defines a good quality of life might be dramatically different from another's definition. No clear boundaries exist between an acceptable versus an unacceptable quality of life for infants. Because of the broad continuum of definitions, quality of life arguments are rarely an ethical "trump card." In fact, although the topic is commonly discussed amongst clinicians, it usually carries little weight in ethical analysis, largely because of the difficulty in pinning down what the "good" is in a "good" quality of life.

Prognostic uncertainty, withdrawal versus withholding treatment, and quality of life are very common topics of discussion in the neonatal setting, but they are also traps that can paralyze productive discussion. Knowing whether some infants will survive or die is difficult. For these infants, continued speculation as to the odds of survival (a 10% chance versus a 20% chance) is unlikely to sway opinion about treatment options. Instead, recognizing that an infant is in the gray zone of uncertainty might help in creating treatment plans that include frequent reassessments of the infant's progress or decline. In this way, providers can monitor when the infant arrives on one side of the gray zone or the other, without wading too long in the bog of uncertainty.

 ## PURPOSE EXERCISE: CONSIDER AND WRITE YOUR ANSWERS TO THE FOLLOWING QUESTIONS

1. What kinds of information might be useful to the team as it contemplates treatment goals for patients in the prognostic "gray zone"?

2. Do nurses have privileged access to any of these kinds of information? How might you contribute to the conversation of Baby G?

Similarly, quality of life arguments are unlikely to be helpful in most situations, as they are too tied to individual perspectives on the goods of living. This is not to say that having frank discussions with parents about possible outcomes is unnecessary; these discussions are essential for respectful, high-quality care. As an aspect of ethics, however, quality of life judgments offer little concrete help. Withholding and withdrawing therapies are viewed by many providers as morally different. Additionally, when treatment withdrawal results in death, some providers and family members might wonder if this action could be considered killing. Providers need to be clear on the fact that removing a treatment that is ineffective is ethically justifiable, and that this action does not constitute killing the patient. The action is identical, morally, to not starting an ineffective treatment in the first place.

When the ethical questions involve whether or not to withdraw treatment, as with Baby G, neonatal nurses will not be the sole decision-maker, but can make real contributions to the decision by being alert to the common traps of becoming too entrenched in uncertainty or quality of life arguments and recognizing (and helping parents and colleagues to recognize) the ethical foundations of withdrawal of ineffective treatments. Additionally, nurses can provide important information about not only subtle clinical changes, but also about parents' understanding of the situation and treatment options, their fears, and their desires. Nurses often have an awareness of the unease that providers feel when bad news must be shared. As a member of the health care team, nurses can offer to be present for those conversations and to support their colleagues during this time, because telling a parent that his or her child will die is a truly difficult task.

Case Study 11.3

Baby boy P is the 35-week-gestation infant of a star player on the city's professional basketball team. The infant was born with Down syndrome and several congenital anomalies. Currently, Baby boy P is intubated and is receiving multiple medications to support his blood pressure in the NICU. The parents and health care team are planning the next steps, which include several staged cardiac and gastrointestinal surgeries. The public has been informed only that the baby was born yesterday afternoon weighing just under 4 pounds and is in the NICU.

The family wants to maintain privacy as they begin to understand the infant's condition and the implications of each procedure he will require. This, however, is difficult, because the NICU does not have private rooms and the father's visits are obvious (he is over 7 feet tall and is well-known in the city). Further, daily rounds routinely include parents and are conducted at the bedside. Thus, many parents are often in the unit, waiting for their turn in rounds.

Bits and pieces of Baby P's health status have been leaked to the press. Two weeks after his birth, Baby P undergoes his first cardiac surgery. The procedure goes well, but the baby suffers a devastating stroke during his recovery. The health care team and parents have discussed on several occasions the issue of withdrawing aggressive therapies. The news of Baby P's stroke and the topic of withdrawal have spread quickly. Two sets of parents have approached Baby P's parents, saying, "You can't withdraw treatment on your baby. That would be killing him." The parents return to the bedside and ask the nurse if this is true. The nurse reassures them that it is not the same as killing him and that, under difficult circumstances such as these, it is an appropriate option. Nonetheless, the parents leave the bedside deeply disturbed by the other parents' intrusion of privacy and insensitive words.

In this situation, no apparent ethical conflict is occurring in terms of treatment decisions. The parents and health care team are in agreement about the tragic nature of Baby P's condition and are focused on doing what is best for him, regardless of the difficulty of the decision. Instead, the ethical issues here are those of confidentiality, privacy, and advocacy, and these are issues that nurses encounter every day.

Confidentiality and Privacy

Maintaining confidentiality is one ethical obligation of nurses and other health care providers. They are entrusted with delicate, highly personal information and are called upon to respect that the information is being shared to ensure high-quality, appropriate care. In Baby P's case, unit procedures involve daily rounds with parents. At first glance, the health care team does not seem to have breached confidentiality, but this family is particularly vulnerable to gossip-seekers and to curious onlookers. Actions to address the attention this family receives could include pulling a curtain around the bed, asking all involved in rounds to keep their voices low, or conducting rounds in a private room or a more private space in the NICU—all of which can be nurse-driven.

PURPOSE EXERCISE: CONSIDER AND WRITE YOUR ANSWERS TO THE FOLLOWING QUESTIONS

1. Should the standards and practices of confidentiality be different when the parent or patient is well-known to the community?

Privacy allows for time and space to discuss, contemplate, and be with the patient. Similar to confidentiality, privacy involves keeping information away from those who do not need it. Unlike confidentiality, privacy involves a physical space component that is critical. Baby P is in a NICU that lacks private rooms. Because of the father's physical size and well-known persona, his every visit challenges the health care team's attempts at ensuring privacy. Is the nurse's obligation to provide privacy more important in instances where those involved are well-known? Perhaps the obligation is not more important, but certainly is a bit more challenging. What is the nurse's obligation in such a circumstance? In this case, providing the greatest possible degree of privacy during parent visits might mean considering the use of privacy curtains and moving the infant to a more private space (an isolation room, for example, or an area of the unit with less traffic).

Advocacy

The American Nurses Association (ANA) Code of Ethics (2008) contains nine provisions for ethical conduct of nurses. Provision 3 describes the ethical obligation to serve as an advocate for patients. In neonatal nursing, the nurse advocates for two parties: the infant and the family. What does advocating for an infant or family mean? For Baby P, perhaps advocating means making sure he is comfortable and receives high-quality nursing care, and that his parents are well-aware of the problems he faces so that they can make good decisions for him. For Baby P's parents, advocacy could include providing information for them, promoting their privacy, maintaining confidentiality, and speaking up for them against well-meaning but inappropriate comments that challenge the parents' judgment.

Some nurses are comfortable advocating in all of these ways. Others are much less so. Nurses who are less willing to confront poor behavior might find a creative way to advocate for parents. Standing up, however, is an integral part of ethical nursing. Few are comfortable with confrontation, but if the parents understand that the nurse is on their side, advocacy can successfully occur in a variety of ways. The nurse's responsibility is to identify how they are willing to advocate and to carry this through.

> ### Case Study 11.4
>
> Baby girl S was a large-for-gestational-age term infant born after several hours of difficult labor. She was floppy and pale on delivery and required a brief but significant resuscitative effort. She was admitted to the NICU for observation and evaluation. Several hours after her admission, she had increasing difficulty maintaining adequate saturations. Her chest x-ray was suspicious for pneumonia, and she was started on antibiotics. At 18 hours of life, she suffered a pneumo-thorax and required chest tube insertion. Prior to inserting the chest tube, fentanyl was ordered. Unfortunately, too large a dose was given. Baby S suffered chest rigidity, requiring emergent treatment and a brief period of intubation. Fortunately, she recovered without great difficulty. Tara, the resident, and Sue, the nurse, discussed whether or not the parents should be told. Tara refused to tell them what had happened, because the infant recovered and suffered no long-term effects. Sue believed strongly that the parents should be told, regardless of the lack of long-term harm. She said, "If something like this had happened to my baby, I would want to know." Still, Tara refused, stating, "Why tell them? They'll lose confidence in us, and they might even sue us. Medication errors happen sometimes. This was one where all's well that ends well."

PURPOSE EXERCISE: CONSIDER AND WRITE YOUR ANSWERS TO THE FOLLOWING QUESTIONS

1. When have you encountered issues with truth-telling?

2. What was your response?

3. How might you support honesty and openness in your practice?

4. Why is this important?

This case involves at least two ethical issues: truth-telling and fidelity. Embedded, too, are potential issues of incompetence and poor practice patterns. Though the mistake could have been just that, it could also reflect lack of knowledge or ability. If this does indeed highlight a situation of incompetence, then future patients are at risk. The implications of revealing the mistake are greater than they might seem at first glance.

Truth-Telling

The past several years have seen growing support for revealing medication and other errors to patients and families. Such situations are now viewed as opportunities for closing gaps in practice processes, for learning from mistakes, and for fostering trust and confidence with patients and families. Still, the act of disclosure can be frightening and threatening. With the disclosure of error comes a process of investigation into how the mistake was made and the steps needed to prevent this type of error in the future. The abilities of the providers might be revealed during this process, and one of the steps might be ensuring that the entire staff is educated on procedures for giving medications, such as opiates, in the case of Baby S.

Baby S's nurse recognizes that not telling the parents is ill-advised, but cannot convince the resident that this is the appropriate step to take. What is the next step here? To let the issue go? After all, Baby S did recover quickly and shows no signs of harm. Although this is the easiest solution, it is not an appropriate one. It does not allow the nurse to have a clear conscience, threatens the integrity of the provider-parent relationship, and possibly puts future infants at risk. Instead, the nurse can and should seek guidance and support from the attending physician and/or the nurse manager.

Fidelity

Another ethical issue is that of fidelity (loyalty). To whom is the nurse loyal? The nurse has obligations to the patient (and in pediatrics, to the family as well), to self, to colleagues, and to the institution. If Sue does not pursue the issue of disclosing the medical error, she might rationalize that she is being loyal to the institution or to her resident colleague. Additionally, the family might choose to sue should they learn the truth. Therefore, Sue might see keeping the error a secret as a way of protecting herself, the resident, and the institution. However, this is a false view of fidelity for several reasons.

- First, though the family might bring a suit, honest and open communication is likely to be viewed much more favorably than secrecy by the family and by a court.

- Second, the resident is incorrect in saying that no harm has been done. Although no lasting harm has been done, other harms (such as costs for medications and mechanical ventilation and perhaps a prolonged hospital stay) have been incurred.

- Finally, even if the error was not because of incompetence, the process for medication administration should be reviewed to prevent another similar occurrence.

The four cases described here highlight ethical issues that arise repeatedly in neonatology and neonatal nursing. Neonatal nurses encounter many of these issues in everyday practice. Some are very familiar, such as privacy, advocacy, and fidelity, and resolving these types of issues is in line with the nursing role. Others are less familiar (parental authority, futility) and perhaps less comfortable territory for nurses. However, in each of the preceding cases, regardless of the ethical issues at hand, nurses can make significant contributions to analyzing the situation and to identifying resolutions. One need not be (and most providers are not) comfortable with all of the potential ethical issues that might occur to make a difference. In the following section, a different aspect of ethical conflict is discussed. The nursing role can be extraordinarily helpful here, even when the ethical issues are sticky and awkward.

Clinical and Environmental Factors Influencing Ethically Challenging Situations

The ethical issues described so far in this chapter rarely, if ever, occur out of the blue. Instead, they tend to arise over time. An astute clinician can often "see the writing on the wall." Does this mean that predictable factors tend to trigger ethical conflict? This is the hypothesis in a relatively new field of ethics called "preventive ethics." Preventive ethics posits that some factors, if not attended to, serve to trigger ethical conflict (Forrow, Arnold, & Parker, 1993). These factors are not ethical issues in themselves. Rather, they are clinical and environmental factors—many of which the nurse is trained to understand and recognize well. The recognition of and action on these factors can truly make a difference in either preventing or moderating ethical conflict.

What are some common triggers? In large part, the common triggers have been identified anecdotally through clinical experience and case study rather than through rigorous science. Still, neonatal nurses might agree readily that common triggers include ineffective communication, spiritual beliefs, unrealistic expectations, and provider turnover (inconsistency). Neonatal nurses are likely to identify other triggers, such as infrequent parent contact, lack of medical consensus, and fear of litigation. A comprehensive list is beyond the scope of this chapter. However, three very common triggers, ineffective communication, spirituality, and inconsistent providers, are explored here.

Ineffective Communication

Ineffective communication is one trigger factor that does have some scientific support and that continues to be of great concern to providers and parents. Although recent studies indicate that intensive communication interventions can be helpful (Lilly et al., 2000; Penticuff & Arheart, 2005), Lantos and Meadow (2006) have identified this as a key issue driving neonatal ethics today. A recent study (Meyer, Burns, Griffith, & Truog, 2002) found that parents of children in the pediatric intensive care unit (PICU) were greatly concerned about aspects of communication such as honesty, completeness of the "big picture," and consistency of information. Physicians struggle with judging how much information to provide (especially when the prognosis is uncertain), how to give bad news, how to balance bad news with hope, and how best to involve parents in decision-making (Epstein, 2008; Oberle & Hughes, 2001). Similar to the concerns of parents, nurses' concerns appear to focus on honesty and completeness (and their role in providing information—the lines here can be rather gray), and similar to the concerns of physicians, nurses' concerns appear to focus on how to maximize shared decision-making. These are all valid concerns that occur frequently in neonatalology.

 PURPOSE EXERCISE: CONSIDER AND WRITE YOUR ANSWERS TO THE FOLLOWING QUESTIONS

Think about the most recent patient you cared for where conflict was present.

1. Were any of the triggers identified here present?

2. Were there others? If so, what were the triggers in that case?

Nurses often have a keen sense about whether parents understand or agree with what is being told to them. They have the medical knowledge to understand the clinical picture and recognize when difficult conversations need to happen. If ineffective communication is a trigger for ethical conflict down the road, then nurses are uniquely prepared to recognize it and to take action sooner rather than later. Actions that nurses can take include alerting the medical team when parents do not seem to understand or agree with the treatment plan; determining parents' depth of understanding or why they might not agree; and offering to be a consistent provider for the infant and parents (in this way, the parents recognize the nurse, the nurse gains intricate knowledge about the situation, and the nurse is recognized by the team as a point contact for information and ideas).

Spirituality

Parents are sometimes called upon to make difficult decisions for their ill newborns. To do so, they use many angles to arrive at what they believe is the best decision, including consultation with family, discussion with providers, cultural influences, past experiences, and their spiritual beliefs. Although not directly an ethical issue, spirituality contributes to ethical decision-making in profound ways. Many parents draw upon their spirituality for comfort, hope, and support. The topic can be an uncomfortable one for providers to broach, however, because they feel unskilled in dealing with spiritual matters, or they hesitate to squash the hopes and beliefs of parents at exactly the time when parents need something from which to draw strength. Still, acknowledgement of its importance in parents' lives and the decision-making process is an important aspect of maintaining a good relationship with parents. A good relationship, in turn, serves to ease the decision-making burden from parents and providers alike and allows for the possibility of growth and understanding.

A common trigger of ethical conflict occurs when deeply religious parents state that they are "waiting for a miracle" and this is not adequately responded to by providers. Providers need to understand that "miracle" means different things to different people, that challenging parents' beliefs is unlikely to be successful, and that respectful conversations are essential (Delisser, 2009). If nurses recognize that spiritual beliefs present a real or potential barrier to the provider-parent relationship or to decision-making, they can take several actions.

- First, learn the parents' definition of a miracle, how influential the parents' spiritual beliefs are in the decisions they are making, and what the nursing staff can do to help support them.

- Second, acknowledge the importance of their spiritual beliefs in situations such as these.

- Third, seek professional guidance (such as from hospital chaplains).

- Fourth, pass the information gained to the rest of the health care team.

- Finally, if they have similar religious or spiritual beliefs, serve as a liaison between parents and providers, even if they do not take on a primary role in the infant's care.

List excerpted from Delisser, 2009

These actions show respect for parents' beliefs but do not allow them to trump ethical decision-making. They educate providers about beliefs but do not necessarily require those without training in religion/spirituality to enter into awkward conversations.

Provider Inconsistency

Family-centered care involves respecting parents' dignity, culture, values, and beliefs; sharing information; encouraging participation in decision-making; and collaborating effectively (Institute for Family-Centered Care, 2008). Embedded in all of these components is provider consistency. Parents are deluged with information from every angle (nurses, unit physicians, specialists, nutritionists, physical therapists, and the list goes on and on). Synthesizing this information and making sense of it under stressful conditions are greatly challenging to parents of an ill newborn. When providers have differences of opinion, give multiple options for treatment regimens, or communicate information poorly, many parents are unable to make good decisions for their infants, regardless of their willingness to try. Further, parents need to see familiar faces—those whom they can trust and recognize as lifelines in a busy, chaotic, and frightening unit. Many parents feel as though a consistent cohort of nurses not only fosters a good nurse-parent relationship, but also improves the quality of infant care, because those nurses know the infant well and can detect subtle changes in the baby's condition (Epstein & Baernholdt, 2011).

For infants whose clinical pictures are particularly complex or who are expected to be hospitalized for an extended period of time, striving to identify a small cohort of nursing staff who can take on the bulk of the infant's care on most days might be a critical step in reducing the incidence of ethical conflict. Plenty argue against such a cohort: What if the nurse and family do not get along? What if the nurse feels over-burdened? How are all 24 hours covered by a small number of nurses over a long hospitalization? Professionalism, creativity, flexibility, and planning are certainly necessary in negotiating these issues. They are insufficient, however, to derail the process or to dismiss efforts to improve provider consistency altogether.

The Nursing Role in Ethical Situations

Every team member—physician, nurse, respiratory therapist, pharmacist, nutritionist, social worker, chaplain—has particular ethical obligations to patients and families. Understanding these obligations and being willing to act on them are critical. The ethical obligations of nurses are defined by the ANA Code of Ethics (2008) and include respecting the dignity and worth of every patient; recognizing a primary commitment to the patient; advocating for and protecting the patient; being accountable for one's nursing practice; preserving their own integrity and competence in the field; making a commitment to improve the environment in which nursing care is given; advancing the profession; collaborating with other professionals; and working toward promoting and protecting the integrity of the profession. Given these obligations, not taking action in situations of impending or actual ethical conflict is difficult to justify. At the same time, nurses vary in their ability to take action. Fortunately, nurses can act in many different ways, so any nurse can make real and credible contributions to ethical nursing practice. These actions fall roughly into two categories. First, the nurse can act to prevent ethical conflict. Second, the nurse can act when ethical conflict takes hold.

Acting to Prevent Ethical Conflict

The fact that nurses are present at the bedside 24 hours per day makes nurses uniquely prepared to recognize common triggers of ethical conflict and to act on them before they have an opportunity to fan the flames of ethical conflict. This involves four broad steps.

The first step is improving nursing continuity. Few units subscribe to a primary nursing or team nursing model today. Discontinuity of providers is a barrier against development of a good nurse-parent relationship and might blunt the nurse's ability to identify triggers early. Further, discontinuity weakens the nursing voice when it comes to contributing to difficult decisions. Therefore, one aspect of the nursing role in preventing ethical situations is to lobby for consistent nursing teams, especially for infants whose clinical picture is complicated or whose hospitalizations are likely to be long, or whose parents might be having particular difficulty. In doing so, this cadre of nurses would likely gain the trust of the parents as well as develop unique insight into the situation—allowing for the nurse to a) identify interventions to reduce the impact of a trigger and b) provide a comprehensive and helpful voice in difficult conversations that might take place.

Identifying the common triggers in the unit, and in a clinical situation, is the second step. Several common triggers are described in the previous section, but others certainly exist. Some triggers might be unique to a particular unit (see the following sidebar).

Third, nurses must be ready to act on the identified triggers. Several suggestions are provided for ineffective communication, spirituality, and provider inconsistency. Feasibility is a key component of a successful action. Convening a large group of people, requiring a large commitment of time or resources, or expecting the participation of many people might not be doable on a busy unit. For example, expecting the medical team to draft a daily summary for parents if that is not already in practice is unrealistic. Instead, a focus on what individual nurses can accomplish, at least initially, is more likely to be successful. A time might come when the multitude of professionals working together recognize that addressing triggers is beneficial to the infant, parents, and providers. Then, larger and more substantial steps can be taken for the unit as a whole.

The final step is to evaluate the actions of the health care team. As the hospitalization progresses, determine whether the action taken (that is, the consistent provider group, conversations to better understand parents' perspectives, alerts to other providers that misunderstanding or miscommunication has occurred) appears to have been effective. Does the health care team see the parents' views more easily? Has the parents' understanding of the situation and treatment options improved? Just as the actions to address triggers require some creativity with an eye toward feasibility, so too does the evaluation process. Single actions might be insufficient to address issues, particularly if they are very complicated. A sustained effort might be needed in some cases. Successful interventions should be documented for future use.

Identifying Common Triggers

1. Reflect on past ethically challenging cases with your colleagues. What were the key issues at play?

2. List the problems identified in these situations. Are there any common threads?

3. List the common threads. These are likely to be the most common triggers for a particular environment.

4. Is a similar situation occurring now on your unit? If so, can you see any of the threads that have been identified?

Acting Within Ethical Conflict

What is the nurse capable of and responsible for in ethically challenging cases? One goal of the nurse might simply be to become engaged in the ethical conversations, and not assume that ethically challenging situations are solely for medicine to resolve. This might mean stepping in and advocating for parents who lack understanding, suggesting that physicians have the difficult conversations with parents, calling an ethics consult when necessary, or a host of other actions. Engagement is the first aspect of the nursing role in ethical situations.

Nurses are not expected to analyze or resolve the conflict. Instead, nurses are expected to share specific information or issues helpful to the analysis. The following guidelines might be useful toward that end.

- **Gather information:** Many times, providers feel as if they do not understand fully the issues at hand. Reading the chart and learning about the pathophysiology will be helpful. Ask the physicians and nurses about their perspectives on the issue. Gather different perspectives, especially if no consensus is apparent. What do they see as problems? Talk with family members. What is their understanding of the condition? What is the background of their decision? Who do they draw on for support? What information or knowledge do they appear to be lacking?

- **Identify the ethical issues at play:** This chapter has touched briefly on many of the issues that arise over and over again in neonatal nursing ethics. Best interests, parental authority, futility, withholding versus withdrawing, quality of life, fidelity, privacy, truth-telling—all of these are ethical issues. Identifying and characterizing the ethical issues at play take practice, persistence, and patience. Utilize available resources whenever possible.

- **Identify the clinical particulars that matter:** Clinical situations almost always involve particulars—details that are unique to the situation and that are essential for understanding—for example, the 23-week-gestation infant who is the product of the parents' third and final attempt at *in vitro* fertilization; the 40-week-gestation infant with meconium aspiration and persistent pulmonary hypertension who is the product of a rape; or the 28-week-infant with multiple congenital anomalies born to a 13-year-old mother. The particulars matter.

- **Encourage interprofessional discourse:** Ethical conflict typically involves multiple people, perspectives, and disciplines. Encourage them to talk to one another. When necessary, consider requesting an ethics consult.

Conclusion

Nursing practice is grounded in ethics. Nursing participation in preventing ethical conflict or in the conflict itself is simply one aspect of the profession and is as important as the concrete nursing skills practiced by nurses every day. In neonatology, the added complexities of patients being unable to speak for themselves, the sometimes astounding ability of a young body to overcome enormous odds, the difficulty that modern society has in dealing with pediatric death and disability, and the pressure on parents to ensure the survival of their children create profound uncertainties and differences of opinion. Neonatal nurses are intertwined in all of this and hold a privileged position as ones who can equally well converse with parents as with medicine. Ethical nursing practice embraces this in-between position. Ethical nursing practice also involves attending to oneself. Recognize that daily exposure to pain, suffering, and death as well as cure, elation, and survival takes resolve, compassion, and caring on deep and life-altering levels. Ignoring situations of conflict or shying away from them serve only to undermine the nurses' ethical practice, moral integrity, and ability to do nursing work well.

Talk About It!

- How will you work to prevent ethical conflict in your unit? What role would you like to play in the ethical aspects of your work? How will you make that happen?

- How do professionals communicate with each other on your unit? How do they communicate with parents? What can you do to improve communication on your unit with other providers and/or with parents?

- What common triggers occur on your unit? Do you recognize them when they occur? How will you act on them from now on?

References

American Nurses Association (ANA), & Fowler, M. D. M. (Ed.). (2008). *Guide to the code of ethics for nurses: Interpretation and application*. Silver Spring, MD. Nursesbooks.org

Beauchamp, T. L., & Childress, J. F. (2009). *Principles of biomedical ethics* (6th ed.). New York: Oxford University Press.

Campbell, A. G., & McHaffie, H. E. (1995). Prolonging life and allowing death: Infants. *Journal of Medical Ethics, 21*(6), 339-344.

Campbell, D. E., & Fleischman, A. R. (2001). Limits of viability: Dilemmas, decisions, and decision makers. *American Journal of Perinatology, 18*(3), 117-128.

Carse, A. L. (1991). The "voice of care": Implications for bioethical education. *Journal of Medicine and Philosophy, 16*(1), 5-28.

Chadwick, J. & Mann, W. N. (1983). *Hippocratic writings*. New York: Penguin.

Council on Ethical and Judicial Affairs, American Medical Association. (1999). Medical futility in end-of-life care: Report of the Council on Ethical and Judicial Affairs. *Journal of the American Medical Association, 281*(10), 932-947.

Delisser, H. M. (2009). A practical approach to the family that expects a miracle. *Chest, 135*(6), 1643-1647.

Epstein, E. G. (2008). End-of-life experiences of nurses and physicians in the newborn intensive care unit. *Journal of Perinatology, 28*(11), 771-778.

Epstein, E. G., & Baernholdt, M. (2011). Application of a primary care continuity measure in the NICU: Implications for end-of-life research [Abstract]. Southern Nursing Research Society 2011 Annual Conference, Jacksonville, FL.

Epstein, E. G., & Delgado, S.H, (2010). Understanding and addressing moral distress. *Online Journal of Issues in Nursing, 15*(3), Manuscript 1.

Forrow, L., Arnold, R. M., & Parker, L. S. (1993). Preventive ethics: Expanding the horizons of clinical ethics. *Journal of Clinical Ethics, 4*(4), 287-294.

Frick, S., Uehlinger, D. E., & Zuercher Zenklusen, R. M. (2003). Medical futility: Predicting outcome of intensive care unit patients by nurses and doctors —A prospective comparative study. *Critical Care Medicine, 31*(2), 456-460.

Fuchs, V. R. (1968). The growing demand for medical care. *New England Journal of Medicine, 279,* 190-195.

Gilligan, C. (1987). Moral orientation and moral development. In E. F. Kittay & D. T. Meyers (Eds.), *Women and moral theory* (pp. 19-33). Totowa, NJ:Rowman & Littlefield Publishers,

Hofman, B. (2002). Is there a technological imperative in health care? *International Journal of Technology Assessment in Health Care, 18*(3), 675-689.

Institute for Family-Centered Care. (2008). *Advancing the practice of patient- and family-centered care.* Bethesda, MD: Author.

Jonsen, A. R., Siegler, M. & Winslade, W. J. (2006). *Clinical ethics: A practical approach to ethical decisions in clinical medicine* (6th ed.). NY: McGraw Hill: Medical Publishing Division.

Kasman, D. L. (2004). When is medical treatment futile? A guide for students, residents, and physicians. *Journal of General Internal Medicine, 19*(10), 1053-1056.

Kopelman, L. M. (2005). Rejecting the Baby Doe rules and defending a "negative" analysis of The Best Interests Standard. *Journal of Medicine and Philosophy, 30*(4), 331-352.

Kopelman, L. M., Irons, T. G., & Kopelman, A. E. (1988). Neonatologists judge the Baby Doe laws. *New England Journal of Medicine, 318*(11), 677-683.

Lantos, J. D., & Meadow, W. L. (2006). *Neonatal bioethics: The moral challenges of medical innovation.* Baltimore, MD: The Johns Hopkins University Press.

Lilly, C. M., De Meo, D. L., Sonna, L. A., Haley, K. J., Massaro, A. F., Wallace, R. F., & Cody, S. (2000). An intensive communication intervention for the critically ill. *American Journal of Medicine, 109*(6), 469-475.

Meadow, W., Frain, L., Ren, Y., Lee, G., Soneji, S., & Lantos, J. (2002). Serial assessment of mortality in the neonatal intensive care unit by algorithm and intuition: Uncertainty and informed consent. *Pediatrics, 109*(5), 878-886.

Meyer, E. C., Burns, J. P., Griffith, J. L., & Truog, R. D. (2002). Parental perspectives on end-of-life care in the pediatric intensive care unit. *Critical Care Medicine, 30*(1), 226-231.

Oberle, K., & Hughes, D. (2001). Doctors' and nurses' perceptions of ethical problems in end-of-life decisions. *Journal of Advanced Nursing, 33*(6), 707-715.

Penticuff, J. H. (1998). Defining futility in neonatal intensive care. *Nursing Clinics of North America, 33*(2), 339-352.

Penticuff, J. H., & Arheart, K. L. (2005). Effectiveness of an intervention to improve parent-professional collaboration in neonatal intensive care. *Journal of Perinatal and Neonatal Nursing, 19*(2), 187-202.

Truog, R. D., Brett, A. S., & Frader, J. (1992). The problem with futility. *New England Journal of Medicine, 326*(23), 1560-1564.

United States Department of Health and Human Services (USDHHS). (1985). Nondiscrimination on the basis of handicap relating to health care for handicapped infants. Procedures and guidelines, final rule. *Federal Register, 50,* 14879-14892.

van Zuuren, F.J., & van Manen, E. (2006). Moral dilemmas in neonatology as explained by health care practitioners: A qualitative approach. *Medicine, Health Care and Philosophy, 9,* 339-347.

Weir, R. (1984). *Selective nontreatment of handicapped newborns: Moral dilemmas in neonatal medicine.* New York: Oxford University Press.

PEDIATRIC ETHICS: WHAT MAKES CHILDREN DIFFERENT?

12

–Lucia D. Wocial, PhD, RN
Nurse Ethicist, Indiana University Health
Adjunct Assistant Professor
Indiana University School of Nursing

Think About It!

- Children may not be adults, but nurses owe them the same obligation of respect.

- Children should be allowed the opportunity to participate in decisions about their own health care.

- Nursing caring behaviors can promote parents' trust and confidence that they are doing the right thing for their children.

- The close relationships nurses form with children and their family are central to nurses' role in addressing ethically challenging situations in pediatrics.

Children are not miniature adults. They face different types of illnesses, have an incredible capacity for recovery, and are not considered fully independent autonomous agents. First and foremost, it seems unnatural to consider that children get serious illnesses or die. We tend to view children as innocents and so feel that any illness or harm that comes to them is somehow unfair. (Jecker & Pagon, 1995). Life-threatening injury and illness in childhood create intense emotional burdens on those who are charged with making decisions for those children, compounding the ethical challenges in these circumstances. The relationships among children, their parents, and those who care for them add another layer of complexity to the ethical issues in pediatrics.

For adults, decisions about appropriate medical care hinge largely on autonomous choices and informed consent. Because the capacity of children to make decisions for themselves develops over years, children must have someone make decisions for them. The decision-makers are typically parents; however, health care professionals have a special obligation to consider the interests of children independently from decisions their parents make. Children might not be independent, autonomous agents, but respecting them as people demands that we consider their preferences, within the context of their developmental abilities and the nature and seriousness of whatever illness they face. Pediatric ethics' central concern is finding and maintaining the delicate balance between protecting the interests of children and nurturing their capacity to eventually make independent choices in their own best interest.

Unexpected Acute Illness in Children

Children are more likely than adults to experience an acute episode of illness. According to the Centers for Disease Control and the National Center for Health Statistics, unintended injury is the leading cause of death in children older than 12 months. Table 12.1 details the leading causes of death for children, broken down by age category (CDC, 2011). The leading causes of death in infants are congenital anomalies and prematurity. For toddlers, the leading causes of death are nonaccidental injury, congenital anomalies, and homicide. For children ages 5-9 years, accidents, cancer, and congenital anomalies are the main causes. Between the ages of 10 and 14 years, accidents, cancer, and suicide lead the list, and for children more than 15 years old, accidents, homicide, and suicide, with cancer a close fourth, are the leading causes of death. In contrast, the leading causes of death for adults are chronic illnesses, such as heart disease. Even though children on the whole use fewer health care resources than adults, the per unit cost of an individual child's care is often higher. In other words, when children are sick, they are really sick (see Table 12.1).

Table 12.1   Causes of Death in Children in the United States

Age (years)	Cause of Death (Descending order)
Up to 1 year	1. Congenital malformations, deformations and chromosomal abnormalities 2. Prematurity 3. Sudden Infant Death Syndrome 4. Newborn affected by complications of pregnancy 5. Accidents
1-4	1. Accidents 2. Congenital malformations, deformations, and chromosomal abnormalities 3. Malignant neoplasms 4. Assault/homicide 5. Diseases of the heart
5-9	1. Accidents 2. Malignant neoplasms 3. Congenital malformations, deformations, and chromosomal abnormalities 4. Assault/homicide 5. Diseases of the heart
10-14	1. Accidents 2. Malignant neoplasms 3. Congenital malformations, deformations, and chromosomal abnormalities 4. Intentional self-harm 5. Assault homicide

Age (years)	Cause of Death (Descending order)
15-19	1. Accidents 2. Intentional self-harm 3. Assault/homicide 4. Malignant neoplasms 5. Diseases of heart

Data from National Vital Statistics Report, Vol 59, No 8, August 26, 2011. Deaths: Leading Causes, 2007.

Taking Childhood Development Into Account

Between birth and adolescence, children go through tremendous changes. As children change, they typically achieve milestones in their physical, psychological, and emotional characteristics. Illness may have a profound impact on children's ability to achieve these important goals on their journey from being a dependent person to an independent adult.

Physical Developmental Changes

When all goes well, children transform from newborns, totally dependent on others for all physical needs, to adults, totally independent of others in all physical needs. In the first 5 years, a child's metabolism is rapid, with extensive growth. After a slowing, adolescence brings rapid growth that is more maturational than size-related. Before maturation, a child's organ systems go through distinct developmental stages that affect both illness and treatment. The care children require varies not just with their physical growth but also with their developmental needs.

Cognitive Developmental Changes

In ethics, words matter tremendously. For children, this is especially true. Words can be confusing. Some words have different meanings or are heard differently because children do not have the same context as adults. For example, when children hear that they will need an "IV," they might believe they are going to get some "ivy." A "CAT" scan for children might mean they will be visited by a kitty cat. Health care providers who take care of children must carefully avoid potentially ambiguous language. Children, like adults, should always be given the opportunity to share what they understand of information that has been presented to them.

Children's concept of illness can be matched to Jean Piaget's stages of cognitive development (Mahowald, 1993). Roughly speaking, cognitive development begins with prelogical thinking, which is characteristic of children between 2 and 6 years; continues with concrete logical thinking, which is manifest in children between 7 and 10; and eventually progresses to formal logical thinking, which is typical in children who are 11 years and older.

Children who have prelogical thinking are oriented to the here and now and have difficulty conceptualizing time. Fantasy (how they want things to be) influences how they think about things. At this stage, explaining how a virus causes chickenpox is less valuable to a child than learning that red, itchy spots are going to appear. Children in this phase learn by playing, so watching children play is a good way to assess their understanding of what illness means to them and how they understand treatment.

Children who have reached the stage of concrete logical reasoning can generally distinguish between what is internal and external to them. They can think about abstract concepts. Children in this phase learn by asking questions and having an opportunity to explain their understanding of things. At the stage of formal logical thinking, children can point to the source of illness within the body, even while describing an external agent as its ultimate cause. At this stage, they can consider hypothetical situations in relation to themselves. How children think has a profound impact on how health care providers need to communicate with them about illness. The specific age at which each child achieves a particular level of cognitive reasoning varies, and illness can have a significant impact on cognitive development.

Children who suffer from chronic illness such as diabetes or who experience illnesses such as cancer might develop a maturity beyond their years. This maturity suggests that even at younger ages, these children might be better able to handle the full truth of their illness and participate more fully in discussions about treatment options than adults assume they can. The illness experiences that these children have often profoundly impact their quality of life and give them insight into what they think is in their own best interest. Uncertainty and subjectivity will always be part of the equation when considering how best to care for seriously ill children (Buchanan & Brock, 1989).

Uncertain Future

Children have an incredible capacity to recover from illness and injury, but it is not limitless. Uncertainty about the response of a particular patient to treatment always exists because of individual biological variability and because of varying expertise of care providers. Thus, the actual outcome of a proposed treatment for a particular patient always depends upon circumstances of person, places, times, and cultures. The uncertainty is often compounded because very sick children typically suffer from multiple medical problems.

When faced with a choice where some degree of risk exists, we expect the rational person to select the options to maximize benefit and minimize risk. In situations where the risk and benefits to be achieved are uncertain, decision-making is more profound. We have no single rule to follow that can optimize the benefit and minimize the harm in uncertain circumstances. In situations of uncertainty about the outcome of medical interventions, despite the obvious emotional burden, parents should be supported and encouraged to remain intimately involved in the decision-making process about treatment choices for their children.

Returning children to their state of health prior to an injury or illness can be deceptive, because restored health in the short-term might offer few clues about long-term outcomes regarding quality of life and evolving autonomy. This problem is compounded by the amount of time it takes to know if interventions have worked. For example, take an infant whose major developmental markers are eating, sleeping, crying, urinating, and having bowel movements. It takes very little brainstem to do these tasks. It might take years before it becomes clear that the "healthy" baby and her family are going to face significant challenges such as learning disabilities, developmental delays, cerebral palsy, blindness, or deafness. No matter how good the diagnostic test, the physicians, or the institution, establishing a prognosis for a child has inherent uncertainty.

For adult patients, health care providers recognize and for the most part accept that some situations might be "worse than death." These situations are typically based on assessments of quality of life, which is a very subjective standard. When adults express a treatment preference in conflict with recommendations from the health care team, those preferences must be respected. When adult patients are not capable of making decisions, a surrogate must make decisions for them.

If surrogates' decisions are contrary to recommended treatment, surrogates have the burden to provide some evidence for how the decisions, including the impact they will have on the patient's quality of life, are consistent with adult patients' values and preferences. Surrogates for adults have some opportunity to discover preferences because, for the most part, adults live as independent moral agents, and surrogates can draw inferences about adults' preferences from how they live their life. For children, this is not so because they, by definition, have limited life experience. Knowing what is important to a child depends in large part on the child's family situation. Assessments about whether or not a situation for a child is "worse than death" are much harder to reconcile.

Paternalism: Looking Out for Children

Doing good for others, the act of being beneficent, is a hallmark of health care. In its most general form, the principle of beneficence establishes an obligation to confer benefits and actively prevent and remove harms. Paternalism—relying on one's own judgment to determine what is best for a patient—might be considered the ultimate application of the principle of beneficence. Paternalism is a behavior and an attitude that seek to protect another person by promoting the autonomy of that person and, when necessary, by overriding that person's autonomous choices to do what the protector believes is best for that person (Mahowald, 1993). Parents do this for their children daily, whether by setting a consistent curfew or insisting that children eat vegetables or do their homework. However, when the decisions are related to chemotherapy for leukemia or a tracheostomy for respiratory support, those everyday paternalistic decisions seem trivial in comparison.

Parents have obligations to ensure survival, to mitigate or prevent pain, and to respect and encourage the developing autonomy of their children. As children grow and develop, parents are challenged to support their emerging capacity to make decisions for themselves, while still protecting them from significant, preventable harm resulting from unwise choices (President's Commission, 1983). Few of us would want anyone to intrude on how we parent our children, yet when a child is sick, health care professionals have a primary beneficent obligation to children in their care, which at times might cause them to challenge a parent's decision about what is best for the children. This challenge should happen only when serious disagreements about what would be in a child's best interests exist and when a failure to question the parents' decision would put the child at risk for significant harm.

In the pediatric setting, multiple issues profoundly impact considerations of doing anything less than "everything" for a child: the inherent uncertainty of treatment outcomes, a child's capacity for recovery, the reluctance of adults to accept the death of a child, and the subjectivity inherent in quality of life assessments. Because children are so vulnerable, until parents clearly have a complete understanding of treatment options, in general, children receive all available life-sustaining treatments. Combine this with health care providers who are unwilling or unable to face what they perceive as defeat, and over time the default position on what is in the children's best interest has become full, aggressive, life-sustaining treatment in all cases, for all patients.

Best Interest: A Guide to Doing What Is Right

The concept of best interest represents a positive obligation—a duty to do what best promotes someone's interests, or is most conducive to his or her good. At different periods in history, and within different cultures, opinions regarding children's best interests have varied. Adding to the difficulty of defining what is in someone's best interest is the mistaken belief that one single best interest exists. Best interest is not a literal and absolute commandment; rather, it is a guiding principle (Buchanan & Brock, 1989). Put more simply, no one single best interest exists, and best interest is not objective.

Because best interest includes a whole life perspective, not just a momentary resolution of a problem, no one individual has all the information necessary to determine a patient's best interest. The definition of what is in a child's best interest tends to be paternalistic, and in pediatrics it might easily be confused with determining what the indications for medical treatment are; thus, it is usually heavily influenced by professional medical opinion. Determining best interest depends in part on the framing of information presented to the child and her parents. Providers must be careful to present information as being based on clinical judgment and not simply imply that the information is "the one truth" about a child's condition or treatment (Jecker & Pagan, 1995).

Consider also that children do not exist outside the context of their families. When considering what is best for an individual child, it is crucial to include the family as part of that consideration. Because pediatric health care providers have an independent relationship with children, they are obliged to assess what they believe is in the children's best interest, especially when that determination is at odds with the course of action being advocated by parents (American Academy of Pediatrics [AAP], 1995). In circumstances where the health care team and parents are in conflict over what is in a child's best interest, only when great effort has been expended to find a common ground should health care professionals seek legal recourse to resolve the conflict (AAP, 1995).

In the face of conflict, health care providers might be so certain of the correctness of their standpoint that they turn to the legal system for help. However, health care providers need to remember that when that happens, decision-making for the child will be removed from the parents and health care providers. In such cases, judges who have no specific medical knowledge or relationship with the patient become responsible for making the decisions (Johnson, 2009). A legal solution most certainly means the key stakeholders will lose control of the situation. Relationships within the family and among the patient, family, and health care providers might be broken beyond repair, so every effort should be made to avoid legal action.

Case Study 12.1 illustrates the complex challenge pediatric health care providers face when doing what they believe is best for a child comes up against a parenting-style choice.

> ### Case Study 12.1
>
> A is an 11-year-old African-American male with new onset Type I diabetes mellitus. He lives at home with his divorced mother and three younger siblings. He spends time every other weekend at his father's house. His parents continue to have a contentious relationship and communication is challenging. A is an average student but not currently involved in any extracurricular school activities. At the time of his diagnosis, he had lost 10 pounds and was in diabetic ketoacidosis. He spent more than 24 hours in the PICU before being moved to a general pediatric unit.
>
> The philosophy of the medical team is that the adults are responsible for managing the patient's diabetes and not the patient. Both parents were informed that anyone who cares for the patient will need to complete 2-3 days of diabetes education. A would be encouraged to participate in the education as much as he wants, but it will not be required for him at this time. The patient may decide to take on certain tasks related to his daily diabetes care, such as blood sugar testing, but the medical team expects the patient to be supervised in all aspects and for the parents to do the overall disease management.
>
> This family expresses the strong belief that the patient should not only be required to learn all aspects of his care, which will include insulin injections, finger pricks to test blood sugar, recognition and treatment of hypo/hyperglycemia, and carb counting, but also knowing when to contact the diabetes phone nurse for changes in his diabetes plan of care. Parents believe this independence is essential, as the patient is the "one who has to live with the disease, and the sooner he learns how to handle it the better." The medical team has shared its concerns that this is too much responsibility for a child of his age and that the parents need to maintain oversight and offer to help him with certain aspects, or at times, even all of his care for the foreseeable future so that he won't become overwhelmed with such responsibility before he has the maturity, judgment, and decision-making skills to do so. This often is not until late adolescence.
>
> The parents and the team are at an impasse, as the parents insist the patient be taught all skills and that they will be observers. The team refuses to assume this approach, and there is discussion of involving Child Protective Services.

Nurses are largely responsible for educating children and their families about illness and how to manage chronic illness. In this role, nurses must learn to help parents see that a perceived criticism of a parenting approach is instead an application of past clinical experience. Helping families see that for children, managing chronic illness is not the same as learning to do other chores such as clear the table or complete a homework assignment. Nurses can best do this by affirming that parents know their children best as people, but health care providers have more expertise when it comes to learning to manage a chronic illness. Doing this helps reinforce the message that the health care team is first and foremost motivated by concerns for what is best for children.

Quality of Life

Unless we are willing to accept that perpetuating the life of a child is always in that child's best interest, we must address quality of life when considering best interests. Quality of life is a difficult concept to define in a precise way. It is more than physical health. It is a subjective sense of satisfaction that a person experiences related to her or his physical, mental, spiritual, and social situation. How someone evaluates her or his quality of life changes over time and is invariably a highly personal value judgment. Early in children's lives, physical and biomedical factors are used to evaluate quality of life. As children age, however, psychosocial factors become more dominant in how they and their family evaluate their quality of life. One of the most troubling and persistent issues in pediatrics is whether or to what extent the expectation of handicaps and other lifestyle-limiting conditions should be considered in deciding how or whether to treat seriously ill newborns and children.

In the early 1980s, the President's Commission for the Study of Ethical Problems in Medicine and Biomedical and Behavioral Research recommended a very restrictive standard: A decision not to provide life-sustaining treatment based on permanent handicaps can be justified only when they are so severe that continued existence would not be a net benefit. However, how one determines the net benefit in such cases is not clear.

The more time people spend with each other, the more in tune they become with the others' needs (Blustein, 1991). This is especially true for nurses who provide care to sick children. Nurses spend more time with patients than any other member of the health care team, and nurses are often the ones who have the opportunity to explore the values and preferences of children and their parents. They are able to form therapeutic relationships with parents, separate from their relationships with children. In this way, nurses may be uniquely positioned to leverage these relationships and navigate conflict, in some cases avoiding pursuing a legal resolution.

Members of the commission believed that a strict standard should be used for children in part because they are among the most vulnerable patients, and so much uncertainty about their ability to recover from serious illness exists. The standard excludes consideration of the negative effects of an impaired child's life on other persons, including parents, siblings, and society. The guide offered by the commission places a great burden on the physician and might in effect delegate the power to define a satisfactory quality of life and the best interests of the child to the physician.

Over time, many bioethicists in pediatrics have argued that this recommendation has some significant flaws precisely *because* it fails to consider the child in the context of her family. It also favors decisions to pursue aggressive life-sustaining treatment for children, minimizing the importance of the burden that treatment might have on the children and their family. The children and their parents must live with the consequences of difficult decisions in a way that no health care provider could ever truly appreciate. Though it is true that children are taken care of by adults and are not capable of making independent decisions about treatment, children have rights and ought to be considered as more than the recipients of the good will of adults. Children deserve respect, which means they must be included as participants in decision-making processes when possible.

The significant amount of time nurses spend with sick children and their families poses challenges. Nurses are acutely aware of the burden children bear while they undergo treatment, in part because in some cases, even routine nursing care can cause a child significant discomfort. For nurses, this intense exposure to suffering may cloud their judgment regarding how much is too great a burden. Nurses run the risk of becoming too enmeshed with their patients and the patients' families. However nurses must not shy away from expressing concerns when they believe the burden a child faces from treatment may be more than the potential benefit the treatment has to offer.

Informed Consent, Parental Permission, Assent, and Dissent

Bringing a child and her family to an informed understanding of the medical facts and treatment options available can be a complex and difficult process, one which requires consideration of the child and her parents. First, we need to be attuned not only to the children's particular level of knowledge and their ability to absorb, synthesize, and retain information, but also to the fears, anxieties, or special vulnerabilities that might be interfering with the decision-making process for them. The same care must be taken when considering how to share information with the children's parents. This does not require an explicit list of items to evaluate, but attentiveness for relevant details and the skill to bring them forward. Additionally, parents might have distinct attitudes about what and how health care providers should communicate with their children. It is not uncommon for parental preferences in this matter to conflict with health care providers' recommendations, which are naturally a source of tension at a difficult time. Consider Case Study 12.2.

Case Study 12.2

B is a 9-year old girl suffering from acute lymphocytic leukemia (ALL). B's mother has been present in the hospital during the majority of her treatment. B is the middle of three children in her family, and she is particularly close to her 6-year-old sister. Despite aggressive treatment, B's ALL has not responded well to treatment. The medical team feels that B will not survive her illness. B's mother insists that the medical team not discuss B's illness with her. She insists that the health care team remain upbeat.

B often asks her nurse if it would be possible for her younger sister, Sally, to visit. On this particular day, B tells her nurse, "I really want to see Sally before I go." When the nurse asks, "Go where?" B replies that she thinks she will be going to heaven soon.

The nurse caring for B knows that her mother does not want the health care team to talk with B about her illness. However, it is clear that B knows more about her illness than B's mother acknowledges. The nurse caring for B can play a pivotal role in helping B's mother appreciate what B knows and to help the mother understand that B has some emotional issues that need to be addressed, and that these issues can be addressed most effectively if discussed openly. The nurse in this case can diffuse conflict between the parents and the team and help the mother and the team focus on meeting the needs B is expressing.

The American Academy of Pediatrics (AAP) advises practitioners that children should be involved in decisions about their treatment. Involving them in the process does not mean they get the final say as if they were autonomous decision-makers. Nor does it mean that all children must be included in discussions about every aspect of their treatment. However, it does mean we have an obligation to determine how much children want to know about their illness and treatment. In discussions about treatment options, for children, it is less about what they are told and more about what they can understand.

In pediatrics, whether the illness is chronic or acute, we should start with the premise that children are capable to the extent that their developmental age allows them to be. Decisions about what treatments to provide to children should be reached through a collaborative process that includes physicians, nurses, parents, and, to the extent they are able, the children for whom the treatment is being considered. This approach is consistent with the doctrine of informed consent, the central focus of decision-making for adult patients.

Capacity, the ability to make an informed choice, is not an all-or-none concept but rather depends on the question under consideration. If the risks are low, the standard for determining capacity is lower, and vice versa (great risk requires a higher standard of capacity). This is especially true in the care of adolescents. Parents justifiably have authority over their children because they are primarily responsible for raising them, and that responsibility necessitates some authority over decision-making. In general, parents know their children best, and affection and close family ties mean parents will most likely make decisions that are based on the best interests of the children. Apart from the children, parents are the ones who must live most intimately with the consequences of the decisions (AAP, 1995).

Informed Consent

Informed consent is a process designed to help patients freely choose a treatment option that is most consistent with their values and most likely to help them achieve their goals of care. Informed consent depends on a patient's capacity to make a decision. Having capacity means patients can understand information they are given, they can reason about the available options and the consequences of selecting from the options presented, and they can freely choose in a way that is consistent with their core values. The most crucial element in this process, the foundation on which all decisions are made, is the sharing of information.

The information about treatment options should be presented to patients in language they can understand. It should include the nature of the illness, any diagnostic tests needed to determine a recommended treatment option, the probability that such treatment will be successful, any risks and benefits associated with the recommended treatment option, and any alternative treatments, including no treatment and the corresponding likelihood of success, risks, and benefits. Table 12.2 highlights some of the key elements of informed consent. The goal of the informed consent process is to help the patient achieve a solid understanding of the clinical situation and arrive at a choice about treatment in a timely way.

Table 12.2　Elements of Informed consent

Capacity to make decisions	Ability to understand the situation as well as information presented Reason through the alternatives presented Communicate clear choices
Reasons for treatment	Diagnosis, tests needed to make a prognosis about disease and treatment options
Treatment options	Risks, benefits of all treatments, including no treatment.

Older children might meet the requirements of informed consent, even if they do not meet the legal requirements of consent. At the other end of the spectrum are the times when the children have no capacity for understanding or providing consent. Participation of young children in health care decisions is mainly a matter of sensitive disclosure. Even at an early age, most children have at least a rudimentary understanding of basic concepts such as sickness and health. Using clear, age-appropriate communication demonstrates respect for children's developing autonomy and fosters a sense of cooperation and collaboration, which in turn can have a positive influence on efforts to obtain their agreement to accept treatment. (AAP, 1995)

When seeking a child's cooperation in treatment, health care providers' obligation to disclose information to children is proportionate to both the likelihood that the children will understand the information and the risk of harm from the disclosure. Truth-telling is essential when disclosing information; it is the foundation of informed consent. Being truthful with children and their parents fosters trust and helps them cooperate with treatment and cope with and recover from illness. Generally, what children imagine might happen is worse than hearing an accurate description of what they can expect. Likewise, being untruthful about what a child can expect (for example, "this won't hurt") violates children's trust. Lying to children is not ethically defensible.

Sometimes, disclosing information to children might lead to significant resistance from the children. In circumstances where disclosure poses harm to the children, it is justified to withhold information, but not to be untruthful. Though disclosure is a component of respect for autonomy, it is not equivalent to the obligation of obtaining assent, or respecting dissent, after disclosure is provided. For example, a 7-year-old's assent is not required for a lumbar puncture (LP) if the procedure is necessary for diagnosis of meningitis. However, the same child might decide whether to present her left or right arm for a blood sample. Because pediatric patients cannot consent, their parents are their surrogate or proxy decision-makers. Informed consent is specific to the individual patient, so in pediatrics, parents are providing informed permission rather than consent.

Parental Permission

Parents have extensive authority over decisions for their children, but it is not absolute and, in some cases, their legal role might be unclear (for example, divorced and blended families). Parents who face a difficult treatment choice for their children struggle with hope, fear, and grief. It is tough to think clearly in the midst of these intense feelings. Yet, no matter what information they receive or whose advice and counsel they seek, ultimately, parents are left with the decision. In giving informed permission, parents should expect to experience the same informed consent process they would experience if they were the patient. Because parents and health care providers both have obligations to a sick child, decisions about treatment options should be shared and focused on determining the best interests of the child. In a pluralistic society with many diverse religious and cultural practices, coming to consensus on what is in children's best interest can sometimes be problematic, particularly as children approach adolescence and begin to develop their own core values and preferences.

Assent

Children might not be able to consent, but including them in the decision-making process shows them respect and nurtures their emerging capacity as decision-makers. The AAP has identified four key elements in the assent process:

1. Helping children achieve a developmentally appropriate understanding of the nature of their condition

2. Telling the children what they can expect with diagnostic tests and treatments

3. Evaluating the children's understanding of the information shared, including an assessment of whether or not the children are feeling inappropriate pressure to undergo treatment

4. Asking the children for their willingness to accept treatment

In asking children about treatment, the provider and parents should seriously consider the children's preferences. To ask with no intention of considering the children's preferences would only serve to undermine the trust the children have in both their parents and those taking care of them. In certain circumstances children must undergo treatment, even if they object. In the spirit of assent, the children should be told this fact, rather than be presented with a false choice. Consent, permission, and assent are particularly challenging concepts to honor when caring for adolescent patients.

The Society for Adolescent Medicine endorses a strong position favoring protection of confidentiality when caring for adolescent patients (Society of Adolescent Medicine [SAM], 2004). This approach is particularly challenging in part because health care providers have separate and distinct relationships and obligations to adolescent patients and their parents. Parents often have difficulty accepting that at some point, the health care provider will not disclose details about their children's treatment without the children's permission. Successful application of this approach depends on open conversations with adolescents and their parents, individually and together. The position is consistent with acknowledging the development of maturity for adolescents and the reality that without confidentiality and privacy protection, adolescents might fail to seek essential health care related to sensitive issues such as sexually transmitted diseases, contraceptive care, outpatient mental health services, and outpatient substance abuse services. Many states allow adolescents to consent to these services without parental involvement (SAM, 2004).

Failure to protect privacy or honor confidentiality of adolescent patients has the potential to cause real harm because of the violation of trust felt by the adolescent. Broken trust might extend beyond the individual who violated the trust to health care providers in general and thus contribute to the likelihood that adolescents will refrain from seeking help. Protecting adolescents' confidentiality and privacy does not extend to situations where a greater good might be served by the disclosure, such as when adolescents are suicidal or homicidal, have life-threatening chemical dependence, or have an eating disorder. However, breaking confidentiality because a provider feels it "is best for the patient" without a strong reason is an inappropriate application of paternalism (SAM, 2004).

Dissent

Children might refuse treatment in some situations. The most obvious is when children have been emancipated from their parents. Criteria for emancipation vary from state to state, but in general, children must be self-supporting, not living at home with parents, and might be married, pregnant, in the military, or declared emancipated by a court. For nonemancipated minors, when the treatment is not essential for the children's well-being or carries great risk, children's refusal might carry significant ethical weight, even if the children cannot legally give consent. In such situations, thinking of a child's "no" when asked to agree to treatment as a "no, not yet" is helpful, meaning health care providers are obliged to continue providing information and to seek an understanding of the reasons for the refusal.

For example, a 15-year-old girl with severe scoliosis refuses to undergo surgery to prevent respiratory compromise. If the girl's parents consent to the surgery, technically, the surgery could go forward even over the objections of the girl. What should be done when she is taken to the OR, screaming, "Don't do this to me!"? The surgical staff could physically or chemically restrain her and perform the surgery. However, though this might achieve the short-term goal of performing the surgery, such actions show complete disregard for the young lady's personhood. If instead the "no" is considered as a "no, not yet," plans for surgery should stop. In a case such as this, a nurse could make a significant difference in this young patient's life. The advocate role of nurses should compel any nurse in this situation to speak up and insist that at the very least, the surgery be delayed so that there may be an opportunity to enlist the patient's co-operation in the procedure.

Using this approach, the health care professionals can acknowledge the girl's feelings and preferences and begin a process of negotiations. Over time, a physician might explain that the girl might die within the next few years if she does not have the surgery. In this case, refusal cannot be honored; however, the child might be given some control over the process. For example, she could choose when to have the surgery, as long as it occurred within a brief window of time. Granting some control might result in the child giving assent to the surgery. In times of refusal, benevolent persuasion is encouraged, and coercion should be used only as a last resort and only when the treatment offers a clear benefit to the child's well-being.

This process of collaboration and negotiation works quite well in situations where consensus exists among the key adult players. However, when the key adult players have conflict, as is the case in many ethically challenging situations, the stakes in pediatrics are very high. The most distressing situations for professional caregivers occur when parents want to refuse recommended treatment, when they insist on treatment that offers no clear benefit and has significant burden, or when children refuse treatment their parents want them to have.

Capable adult patients can refuse treatment recommendations from physicians, even in situations where the refusal will lead to the patient's death. Parents, as proxies for their children, are not as free to refuse recommended treatment, in part because health care professionals have an obligation to children that is separate from the obligation they have to children's parents. Likewise, in situations where parents demand "futile" treatment, providers must consider the burden to the children separate and apart from the parent's demands. Especially in these circumstances, parents and health care providers must balance their tendency to be paternalistic with the children's developing capacity to make informed choices about treatment. Uncertainty, best interest, emotional burden, and paternalism all contribute to a reluctance to consider doing anything less than "everything" to keep critically ill children alive.

When parents or children with capacity refuse treatment, the children, the family, and health care providers all feel a profound impact. When the treatment is considered life-saving, in many cases states have mandated temporary legal guardianship of children so that the children can receive needed medical care. Even in situations where parents claim religious freedom as grounds for refusal, they do not have the right to deny life-saving medical treatment for their children. Refusals based on religious grounds might be considered differently if the child is nearing the legal age for decision-making and the child's refusal is based on her or his own religious convictions rather than those of their parents. However, the majority of cases, after being brought to the attention of a judge, will result in the child being required to undergo a life saving treatment, particularly if the expected benefit is great and the risk of harm is not.

One of the most challenging situations in pediatrics is when children, usually adolescents, refuse recommended medical treatment that their parents want them to have. Considering the children's refusal does not mean it will be honored, particularly in cases where the refusal will likely result in serious permanent harm. However, forcing treatment upon children against their will is a serious situation. Thus, parents and health care providers must weigh the expected effectiveness of the proposed treatment, the burden of undergoing the treatment, and the need for compliance with continued treatment against the practical implications of forcing the treatment on the children (Johnson, 2009).

Consider, for example, a 16-year-old young woman who is receiving treatment for leukemia. Between the third and fourth rounds of chemotherapy, she refuses to allow a lumbar puncture (LP). The procedure is necessary to determine appropriate medication dosing and evaluate effectiveness of the treatment. Her parents say, "Tie her down if you have to," even while the 16-year-old is refusing. Legally, the parents can require that their daughter undergo the treatment. However, the child's form of leukemia is resistant to treatment. Even with the full course of chemotherapy, her chances of survival are 50%. Enduring the chemotherapy requires this very independent, social young woman to remain in the hospital in isolation for a minimum of 4 weeks, and a 20% mortality risk exists with the chemotherapy. Even if treatment is imposed on this child, effectively imprisoning her, the success of this treatment depends on her returning for another round of chemotherapy. Given the limited chance of success, the significant burden and risk, and the practical challenges of imposing the treatment on this child, to override her refusal will most certainly undermine her emerging autonomy and might very likely cause significantly more harm than considering the "no" as a "no, not yet" response and dedicating substantial effort to understand the refusal and negotiate alternatives if at all possible.

When the health care team feels an obligation to honor children's refusal over the objections of parents, the team must be transparent with parents about its reasons and expend every effort to engage the parents and their children in a shared decision-making process. Agreeing to an informed refusal of treatment or setting limits on treatment for children is not any more unethical than setting limits for adults. In many cases, however, it is much, much harder.

Setting Limits

No one likes to consider the possibility that saving children's lives, or offering every available treatment in that effort, is not in children's best interest. But health care is limited in what it can achieve, and the fact that technology exists does not mean it should be used in every case. Clinicians have an obligation to present reasonable options and make a recommendation, not to simply lay out choices and expect family members to choose as if they were ordering dinner. When children experience a life-threatening event, either as a result of an injury, congenital anomaly, or illness such as cancer, parents are commonly involved in an explicit discussion about withdrawing or withholding treatment, sometimes motivated by quality of life concerns and sometimes by futility. Futility can be defined as the failure of a specific intervention to accomplish the goals of care. Using either criterion to consider limiting treatment is challenging because both are subjective.

What should be most influential in these considerations is balancing the suffering children will experience as a result of pursuing treatment against the likelihood of benefit. Intolerable or unbearable suffering typically refers to the physiological burdens or impending death of children and not to the parents' reactions to the children's experience. Likewise, an assessment about children's quality of life must be based on what the children will likely experience, not what someone else might imagine it would be like to live the lives the children might have. The challenge then is to assist parents in focusing primarily on the children, the clinical facts of the case, the reality of the children's suffering, and the limits of medical treatment. When parents consider withdrawing or withholding life-prolonging therapies, health care providers should not consider the situation a failure. In these circumstances, the only "failure" happens when providers fail to provide aggressive symptom management focused on making children as comfortable as possible, allowing them to optimize their quality—if not their quantity—of life. Situations where members of the health care team feel parents are insisting on futile or nonbeneficial treatment are by far the most common of ethically challenging situations in pediatrics. Consider Case Study 12.3 on Baby L.

Case Study 12.3

Born at 23 4/7 weeks gestation, Baby L has spent 6 months in the neonatal ICU. She has experienced multiple complications, including necrotizing enterocolitis, which resulted in the loss of all but 20 cm of her intestines, a grade IV intraventricular hemorrhage, and most recently kidney failure. Her respiratory status has deteriorated, and she now requires significant ventilator support. Her parents have spent time with her every day of the last 6 months. The physicians are now convinced that medical technology cannot even sustain L much longer. Her body is bloated and she has developed significant areas of skin breakdown. When asked by the medical team to consider shifting the goals of care to focus on L's comfort, both parent state, "Don't ask us to make that decision! You have to do everything to save her!" Both parents, however, express concern that L may be suffering. In this scenario, the team may conclude that there is nothing they can do because the parents will not agree to stop treatment.

It is often a nurse who is able to skillfully coax a family to see the suffering of children and the inevitable trajectory of a terminal illness. When nurses invite parents to consider what they would want if children cannot survive an illness, parents may be able to see that sometimes protecting and loving a child means letting go. Nurses may also be in a position to gently but firmly encourage physicians to state simply, but clearly, when saving children is no longer possible, and making them comfortable must be the priority. This approach is one that recognizes parents may wish suffering to stop, but be unwilling or unable to bear the burden of making that decision. This approach allows parents to feel involved in caring for children but not feel ultimately responsible when children die (Paris, Graham, Schreiber, & Goodwin, 2006).

Parents who face difficult decisions, particularly decisions about limiting or stopping treatment that will lead to the death of children, want to believe that the people who are taking care of their children care not just for, but also care about their children. If parents believe physicians and nurses care about their children, they are more likely to trust them. If they trust the physicians and nurses, parents are more likely to believe that limiting treatment is a compassionate choice. Nurses are most often credited with demonstrating caring behaviors when children are sick. Caring behaviors promote parents' trust in the people taking care of their children and confidence in the information they hear and ultimately in the decision they are asked to make (Wocial, 2000).

Advances in medical technology have significantly prolonged the lives of children, even children with complex diseases. However, a longer life (survival) tells only half of the story. A steadfast focus on survival has caused many to negate the impact of life-prolonging therapies on meaningful growth and development of children and the quality of their lives. A growing ethical challenge in pediatrics is the reality that though we might be able to save children from complex illnesses, after they become adults, their access to services and needed medical treatments might be limited because of how the health care delivery system is structured in the United States. For example, children who receive transplants or survive cancer treatments might not be eligible for insurance coverage after they become adults (Kaplan, Green, Balaurie, & Meyers, 2009).

Conflict

The classic definition of an ethical dilemma is a situation where more than one choice is ethically defensible, but the available choices are mutually exclusive, meaning if you pick one, you cannot pick any of the others. True dilemmas in health care are rare, in part because as long as key stakeholders maintain open, honest communication, most conflict can be resolved by negotiating options to achieve a consensus. This is not to say that no conflict exists when it comes to determining how best to care for ill children. Treatment decision conflicts might reasonably trigger an evaluation of children or parents' capacity to make decisions, but these situations should also trigger a reevaluation by the health care team, both of the treatment and of the communication of the recommendation to the family. Unfortunately, no objective formula exists that can incorporate the information about a patient's case and magically arrive at the answer to the question "What should be done?" The element of subjectivity in these cases is irreducible. No advances in prognostic skills, physiology, or even in individual psychology can be expected to eliminate it.

Lessons Still to Be Learned

Ethics in pediatrics is more than issues around death and dying, but those issues are the most poignant and thus have been the focus of this chapter. When serious illness or injury happens to children and their families, it is often an unexpected, traumatic event. Families find themselves forced to trust strangers to act in their best interests. The circumstances are often unfamiliar and even terrifying, and they provide little or no opportunity to develop more than a thin familiarity with the professionals who are to be so entrusted. This awkward reality requires that health care professionals attend more explicitly to the implications of manner, tone, touch, and other forms of demeanor when they communicate.

In modern health care, prestige and praise are seldom afforded to those who accept death rather than pursue any available technology. Health care professionals are applauded for acting, intervening, and forestalling death. In addition, they are naturally optimistic, but this optimism might prevent them from accurate perceptions about the burden of treatment for children. Among the values inherent in modern medical practice are faith in science, a commitment to conquering disease, and forestalling death. The optimism of providers and past experiences with children who beat the odds and recovered from devastating illness can encourage the application of technology to inappropriate levels. Taking care of sick children is intense and highly emotional, which complicates ethically challenging situations. It is a difficult task for anyone to witness the suffering of children without becoming vulnerable. Doing what is ethical in pediatrics requires health care providers to assess as objectively as possible what is in children's best interest and to be exquisitely sensitive to situations where subjectivity clouds their judgment about parents' choices for their children. Professionals who work in pediatrics face a danger of becoming protectors of patients. They inadvertently take on the role of parents, leading to too much involvement with patients or to unjustified paternalism. Health care professionals in pediatrics would do well to establish a firm sense of boundaries and a keen sense of one's own biases. No matter how solid the data, the interpretative filter will always be the health care professional's clinical judgment, which will be colored by past clinical experiences and personal core values. It may be challenging to come to consensus and determine what is in the best interests of a child, but failing to do this powerful reflective work means every child will have to undergo every treatment no matter how painful, or difficult, until such time as the child can speak for herself.

Conclusion

Ethical issues involving children, because they are vulnerable and nurses naturally want to protect them, are especially challenging. As children grow and develop, listening to their values and preferences becomes more critical. However, children develop at their own pace, and there is no way to know exactly at what age they are prepared to be fully engaged in making decisions about their own health care. Identifying what is the right thing to do for children is complicated by the need to form separate relationships with children and their parents. Although parents are ultimately charged with making decisions for children, nurses must be prepared to evaluate what is in children's best interest and advocate for children.

Talk About It!

- What can nurses do to show their respect for children?

- How do you think your own parenting style (or how you were raised if you don't have children) influence how you feel about parents of sick children? How do you expect them to behave?

- Talk with your colleagues about your experiences with critically and chronically ill children. Under what circumstances (if any) would you consider limiting treatments for your own child?

- How close should nurses get to children in their care? To the parents of those children?

References

American Academy of Pediatrics Committee on Bioethics. (1995). Informed consent, parental permission, and assent in pediatric practice. *Pediatrics, 95*(2), 314-317.

Blustein, J. (1991). *Care and commitment: Taking the personal point of view.* New York: Oxford University Press.

Buchanan, A., & Brock, D. (1989). *Deciding for others: The ethics of surrogate decision making.* Cambridge: Cambridge Press

Centers for Disease Control. (2011, August 26). Deaths: Leading causes, 2007. *National Vital Statistics Report*, *59*(8). Retrieved from http://www.cdc.gov/nchs/data/nvsr/nvsr59/nvsr59_08.pdf

Jecker, N., & Pagon, B. (1995). Futile treatment: Decision-making in the context of probability and uncertainty. In A. Goldworth, W. Silverman, D. Stevenson, & E. Young (Eds.), *Ethics in Perinatology* (pp. 48-69). New York: Oxford University Press.

Johnson, C. (2009). Overriding competent medical treatment refusal by adolescents: When "no" means "no." *Archives of Diseases in Childhood*, *94*(7), 487-491.

Kaplan, B., Green, C., Baluarie, J., & Meyers, K. (2009). Ethical challenges in pediatric dialysis and kidney transplantation. In V. Ravitsky, A. Feister, & A. Caplan (Eds.), *The Penn Center guide to bioethics*. New York: Springer Publishing.

Mahowald, M. (1993). *Women and children in health care: An unequal majority*. Oxford: Oxford University Press.

Paris, J., Graham, N., Schreiber, M., & Goodwin, M. (2006). Has the emphasis on autonomy gone too far? Insights from Dostoevsky on parental decisionmaking in the NICU. *Cambridge Quarterly of Healthcare Ethics*, *15*, 147-151.

President's Commission for the Study of Ethical Problems in Medicine and Biomedical and Behavioral Research. (1983). *Deciding to forego life-sustaining treatment: A report on the ethical, medical, and legal issues in treatment decisions*. Retrieved from http://bioethics.georgetown.edu/pcbe/reports/past_commissions/deciding_to_forego_tx.pdf

Society of Adolescent Medicine Position Statement. (2004). Confidential health care for adolescents. *Journal of Adolescent Medicine*, *35*(1), 1-8.

Wocial, L. D. (2000). Life-support decisions involving imperiled infants. *Journal of Perinatal and Neonatal Nursing, 14*(2), 73-86.

REVISITING THERAPEUTIC RELATIONSHIP IN PSYCHIATRIC-MENTAL HEALTH NURSING: TOWARD A RELATIONAL ETHIC

13

–Margaret Cotroneo, PhD, PMHCNS-BC
Emeritus Associate Professor of Psychiatric-Mental Health Nursing
University of Pennsylvania School of Nursing

–Freida Hopkins Outlaw, PhD, RN, FAAN
Director, Youth Health and Wellness Center
Meharry Medical College

–June M. Roman, MSN, RN, PMHCNS-BC
Psychiatric Clinical Nurse Specialist
University of Pennsylvania School of Nursing

Think About It!

- A healing relationship is essential to ethical nursing practice.

- Science and technology are changing the nature of psychiatric-mental health nursing practice

- The nature of practice is changing the way psychiatric-mental health nurses must think about ethics

- In a time of constant change, practice is the living laboratory that shapes and informs ethics.

- The therapeutic relationship is the ethical framework of psychiatric-mental health nursing practice.

The link between quality of health care and quality of life gives rise to some of the most challenging ethical claims of our time. As health care providers, improving the patient's quality of life is our challenge, and providing therapeutic quality of care is our mandate. This mandate shapes professional ethics and comprises the profession's response to social needs, the conduct expected of the professional, and the skills associated with the specific practice of the professional.

For nurses, infusing their relationships with trust is one of their greatest tasks in meeting the ethical claims implicit in the word "quality" and is essential for meeting the professional ethical standards required of all nurses. To honor their commitment of rendering humane, competent, accountable care through the nurse-client relationship, psychiatric-mental health nurses need trustworthy relationships on which they can rely—in families, in workplaces, in communities, in the nation, and in the world. A relational framework for ethics requires an ethical ecology of preserving the resources of relationship by attending to the full context of a therapeutic relationship. This means that the relationship would include not only the nurse-client relationship, but also any other relationships that might be affected during the therapeutic process including the care team, the family, and the community. A relational framework would also include a consideration of the biopsychosocial determinants of health and well-being, cultural and ethnic differences, and consequences of treatment provided by psychiatric-mental health nurses for those who might be affected.

The aim of this chapter is to explore the meaning of the "therapeutic relationship" as the ethical framework of psychiatric-mental health practice and to examine its contemporary applications to better understand its implications for practice in a transforming and evolving health care environment.

Interpersonal Relationships: The Cornerstone of Psychiatric Nursing

In 1952, Hildegard Peplau, considered the "mother of psychiatric nursing," introduced a theory of practice influenced by Harry Stack Sullivan's theory of interpersonal relations. Her theory proposed that the interpersonal relationship is the essence of psychiatric nursing. Nurses, through an intellectual process that is guided by the theory of interpersonal relations, must be aware of the meaning of the interactive process between nurses and patients. In this therapeutic process, nurses are required to understand the meaning of their own behavior when interacting with the patient or their family. This self-awareness developed by nurses was essential to assist the healing of patients. Peplau (1952) proposed that nursing, as a healing art, is inherently therapeutic, with its goal being to help those who are sick and in need of health care. However, to reach this therapeutic goal, nurses and patients have to work together in an interactive process. The therapeutic process might include others, such as the family, but the ethical core of the theory is the commitment to a healing relationship between the nurse and the patient that is inherently interpersonal.

We have seen many developments in relational theory and its application in therapy because of Peplau and Sullivan. The field of health care in general and family therapy and family-oriented primary care in particular have been rich in ethical discourse focused on applications of relationship theory and therapy (McDaniel, Campbell, Hepworth, & Lorenz, 2005). Because of its biopsychosocial orientation, psychiatric-mental health nursing has integrated many of these ideas into the field of practice (Cotroneo et al., 2001). However, though theoretical formulations about the ethics of relationship are readily available, their application to psychiatric-mental health nursing practice requires a continuous dialogue among all of the key stakeholders to remain current. In a constantly changing world, what support and guidance about the ethics of relationship are needed to help psychiatric nurses who are providing care in a variety of settings?

The commitment to relationship has a central place in nursing's code of ethics, both nationally and internationally.

- *Psychiatric–Mental Health Nursing Scope and Standards of Practice* (American Psychiatric Nurses Association and the International Society of Psychiatric-Mental Health Nurses, 2007) posits the foundation of psychiatric-mental health nursing ethics as the therapeutic relationship with the client (p. 51).

- The Registered Psychiatric Nurses of Canada has approved a code of ethics (2010) that clearly identifies the therapeutic relationship as the core of psychiatric nursing practice within a framework of personal responsibility for practice.

- Of the four principal elements identified in the International Council of Nurses (ICN) Code of Ethics (2006), the first states that nurses' primary professional responsibility is to people requiring nursing care.

A reading of these professional codes makes it clear that a healing relationship is inextricably linked to nursing ethics.

In their contemporary practice, psychiatric-mental health nurses and those for whom they care are confronted with an array of treatment choices, stretching the boundaries of knowledge and competence. The decisions that nurses must make in their everyday practice are increasingly more complex, requiring not just a concern for immediate situations that arise but a way of thinking and acting that helps identify real or potential problems. For example, racial and ethnic differences may add to the complexity of relationships between majority caregivers and the patients and families in their care (Institute of Medicine [IOM], 2003). What should psychiatric nurses be aware of when discussing treatment options with ethnically and racially diverse patients and families? Are they aware that their thoughts, feelings, and beliefs about the ethnically or racially diverse patient may affect the options that they offer to the patient and family? This same concern would be operative for psychiatric-mental health nurses when they work with other diverse populations, such as people with physical disabilities and those who have a different sexual orientation. Existing ethical guidelines are indispensable in preventing psychiatric nurses from practicing outside their scope of expertise, but they are only a partial response to the ethical distress that psychiatric nurses might experience in balancing safety, effectiveness, routine tasks, cultural competence, and therapeutic relating in more complex relationships (Ulrich, Hamric, & Grady, 2010).

Case Study 13.1

"Recently, I spoke with a colleague who is working on a legal case. A 45-year-old man was brought into the emergency department after his family reported him missing. He had a history of schizophrenia and was assessed to be a danger to himself and others and was to be admitted to a psychiatric inpatient unit. He was placed in the hall to await admission and eloped from the emergency department. He went home, got his gun, and shot at least one other person and himself. Luckily, no one was killed, but a lawsuit ensued. A psychiatric nurse—who seemed to have done all the right things, except for leaving him alone in the hallway—initially assessed him. Clearly no trusting relationship had been started in this case, and this man had no sense that he could be helped." (J. Roman, Personal communication, August 30, 2011)

What ethically relevant questions arise in this situation and for whom? What actions or behavior would have made it possible to read the context clues in this situation? What kind of relational interventions convey trust and caring to the patient and the family in a stressful environment? What do nurses and other care providers need to engage with the relational context of care?

A Practice Landscape in Transformation

The notion of the centrality of trustworthy relating seems very contradictory in these times of instant, often fragmented and rather disposable connections. People in society are very mobile and dynamic, and increasingly, they are living in a technology-oriented world. Tweeting, blogging, and posting messages on social media sites are the relational networks on which they have come to rely. In this environment, relationships are often matters of convenience and shared interests. In the ethical sphere, this means an even greater emphasis on functionality and effectiveness and a tendency to rely on general ethical principles that apply to autonomous generic individuals. An understanding of context and what motivates, shapes, and sustains individuals, families, and communities seems almost too abstract and inefficient in the resource-constrained environments in which most psychiatric nurses practice. Relationships, however, merit our attention because they have a life beyond any immediate individual consideration—they live on in their consequences for the future and their implications for shaping the quality of our lives and the lives of those to whom our practice commits us. Because of the nature of psychiatric-mental health practice, these commitments have consequences that can extend for many years, in multiple relationships, across generations of a family and a community, and across a range of settings.

With the impetus of the Patient Protection and Affordable Care Act (PPACA; P.L. 11-113, 2010) our health care system is expected to rebalance current acute care models of service delivery. Approaches in which prevention and a concern for the consequences of our actions on quality of life of present and future generations will, out of necessity, be at the center of an evolving health care system. The PPACA identifies great challenges in the management of chronic conditions; primary care (including care coordination, prevention, and wellness); and prevention of adverse events in acute care settings. It envisions a demand for better provision of mental health services, school health services, long-term care, and palliative care (including end-of-life care).

At the center of all of these considerations is the continuous healing relationship. Care coordination, patient-centered care, care partnerships, and population health are terms that are going to be heard over and over again as our systems begin this long period of transformation. Practitioners who can read the signs of the times, who can manage within and across organizations and systems and work in partnerships with patients, families, communities, and with multiple colleagues across disciplines, across settings, and across competencies, are going to be in demand. These activities require the skills of relationship and the ability to read context clues. Moreover, how the health professions will grapple with the ethical implications of the choices inherent in a move toward quality of care is still not clear. For example, if patient-centeredness is a quality measure, what would that look like in terms of patient autonomy?

The ethical concerns might not be so much about individual, autonomous choices as they are about better choices and the effects of choice beyond the individual. The added value to teamwork might not be so much about how well clinicians learn to swim with sharks as it is about how well they learn to swim skillfully with the tide, relying on each other for balance. To confront these challenges, we need courageous problem solvers, not prescribers, creative thinkers, not seekers of the status quo. In this sea of choice and change, it is not enough to ground ourselves as responsible practitioners if we do not have the relational skills to share responsibility with others for the mandated quality outcomes and the ethical decisions they spawn. Relationship is the most important ingredient in any approach to collaboration (Seaburn, McDaniel, Kim, & Bassen(2005). Infusing relationships with trust is going to be our ethical challenge for many years to come, because trust is the ingredient that builds and sustains therapeutic relationships.

The recently released National Prevention Strategy illustrates in diagram the shifting emphasis to quality of life and its challenges (Figure 13.1; National Prevention Council, 2011).

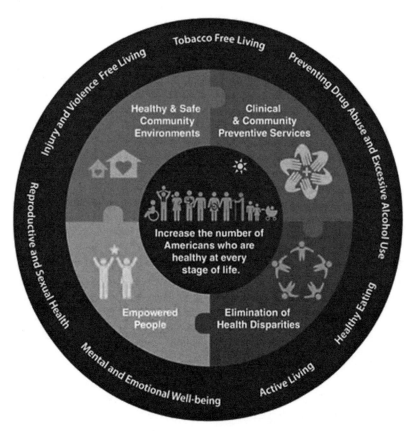

Figure 13.1 National Prevention Strategy: America's Plan for Better Health and Wellness

The emphasis on prevention will have intended and unintended consequences regarding how health care is conceptualized, delivered, and evaluated, and they will extend to all who might be affected by an ethical decision. This fact alone positions relational ethics to play a central role in any health care deliberations.

Relationships, Health Care, and Ethics

During the course of its work, the committee on the Robert Wood Johnson Foundation Initiative on the Future of Nursing at the IOM developed a vision for nursing in a transformed health care system (IOM, 2011). The vision for what would constitute "quality of care" was laid out in at least three earlier reports of the committee (IOM, 1988; 1996; 2001). The committee envisions a future system that makes "quality care accessible to the diverse populations of the United States, intentionally promotes wellness and disease prevention, reliably improves health outcomes, and provides compassionate care across the lifespan" (IOM, 2011, p. 2). In this vision, primary care and prevention are central drivers of the health care system. Interprofessional collaboration, coordinated care, and transparency are the norm. It is also clear that health care has to be delivered in terms that are affordable to individuals and to society.

For psychiatric-mental health nurses to do their jobs, the future demands more complex thinking about ethics, a movement toward a more contextual approach that considers the relational circumstances of action or behavior as well as the behavior itself. Economic drivers might shape the transformations in our health care system, but the important questions nurses are compelled to ask about health and quality of life have to do with how the relationships among patients, family, and nurses will be affected in the evolving environment. Science and technology are changing the nature of practice, and the nature of practice is changing the way we think about ethics, compelling us to be open to new ways of communicating and relating to patients, families, communities, and global interests. Increasingly, our ethical knowledge will be based on our ability to work with "knowledge partners" and to use technology appropriately to help us build and sustain caring relationships.

Complex relationships are driving the health care systems, both nationally and globally. The relationship of genes to the environment and to individual and group health and health outcomes will consume the interest of society well into the future. Genetic relatedness, on account of the newness and potential of the science, has dramatically influenced all other forms of relatedness. The continued advancement of biomedical science as well as the renewed emphasis on the effects of environmental, social, cultural, ethnic, economic, and behavioral determinants on health and quality of life are transforming the systems in which all health care providers, including nurses, practice. Many chronic health conditions that cluster in families result from shared genes, shared social conditions, shared behaviors, and shared environments. Healthy immune function is affected by healthy relationship patterns (Kiecolt-Glaser & Glaser, 1986). Somatic symptoms can serve an adaptive function in the family and be maintained by family patterns of interaction.

Co-occurrence of mental illness with heart disease, diabetes, stroke, or other medical conditions increases clinical risk for patients (Kessler, Chiu, Demler, Merikangas, & Walters, 2005; Pan, 2011). Researchers are challenged to find better ways to explicate the relationships between biology and environment in health outcomes research (Diez Rouz, 2011). On a local, national, and global scale, health disparities and comorbidity are inextricably linked (National Institute of Mental Health [NIMH], 2011).

Because relationships, by their very nature, are dynamic configurations, they require an ethical dialogue that captures, embraces, and bridges evolutions and transformations in both the process and outcome of health care delivery. That kind of dialogue has been emerging in the literature. Interactional concepts such as "shared mind" (Epstein & Street, 2011) have been proposed as a way of balancing individual autonomy with relational autonomy. In relational autonomy, all who are affected by difficult decisions share in the deliberations in an iterative process of "building" a decision. The outcomes of this process might be completely new options that previously had not been identified. Lambert, Soskolne, Bergum, Howell, and Dossetor (2003) extended the notion of fostering autonomy through mutually respectful relationships to public and environmental health. They point out that, as an ethical practice, fostering autonomy means a duty to foster common understanding and "create common knowledge" and not simply provide information and report data (p. 134). From the perspective of moral philosophy, Pettersen (2011) has reconceptualized care as "mature care" that grounds the moral agent in a relational process that is reciprocal and recognizes the interests of both self and others. As a conclusion, he notes that failure to attend to both self-interest and the interests of the person(s) needing care works to diminish responsibility. Spurred by the threat of pandemic influenza, states and local communities have had to grapple with the ethical implications of vaccine allocation, raising questions of transparency, public accountability, proportionality, and risks to autonomy (Thomas & Young, 2011). Harrowing, Mill, Spiers, Kulig, and Kipp (2010) make a compelling case for why it is no longer appropriate to design research in the developing world by applying Western bioethical principles of individual autonomy without also considering the context in which people live and function.

What Is a Relational Ethic, and How Does It Apply to Psychiatric-Mental Health Nursing Practice?

In a time of constant change, practice is the living laboratory that shapes and informs ethics. Relationships are the "working capital" of psychiatric nursing practice—a major resource that not only adds value to the array of biopsychosocial tools available to us but also actually guides and directs them. The economist Robert Reich has described relational capital as the "cumulative trust, experience, and knowledge that forms the core of the relationship between businesses and their customers" (Reich, 2009, p.1).

Nursing is a profession that practices in a business environment. At a time of increased fragmentation of services, more choices and options, and an emphasis on cost containment, the aims of care seem almost contradictory unless one is fully engaged with the resources of care: relationships with clients, families, communities, providers of all kinds, professional colleagues, and policymakers.

The advantages of relational capital are many: getting to know those to whom we offer professional care as individuals and in context of family and community; tracking progress over time; intervening early in problems; tailoring interventions based on evidence; and building relationships of trust on which one can rely for advice and problem solving. The ethics of psychiatric-mental health nursing are not static (role defined) but are shaped by practice, which in turn is shaped by evolving patient and family needs, community requirements, social determinants of health, policy mandates, and evidence. Therefore, beyond technical knowledge and skill and beyond the ethical codes of a profession, we need to reengage with a broader conceptualization of therapeutic relationship.

The word *relational* is subject to many interpretations among ethicists who use it. In general, the person-in-relation to self, neighbor, and the world is posited as the guideline for ethical reflection. Individual moral efforts are given due consideration, but ethical action is understood and interpreted as the consequence of a complex configuration of relating. This configuration is shaped by the give and take of a whole network of relationships that have to be given due consideration.

Traditionally in health care, the motif of responsibility for one's actions has been the organizing principle for ethical action. These responsibilities are attached to individual achievement in the moral effort. They are codified in manuals and statements of individual professional conduct. This individual perspective is understandable and, in some situations in which the ethical choices are clear, it is even desirable. The language of relationship is difficult to translate into the language of ethical norms and behaviors. However, this individual focus has too often led clinicians to a practice shaped by ethical stagnation— ethics divorced from the ever-shifting nature of context and the give and take of relationship over time. The authors define a relational ethic as the human claim on relationship through the simultaneous consideration of the needs, interests, and obligations of all relating partners in a dialogue of fair give and take.

A relational ethic represents another worldview: that of the multiperson system. Standards and qualities derived from personal or group values must always be considered because they are motivational. However, a relational ethic goes further in including concepts, actions, and behaviors; methods of inquiry; and practices derived from the *actual experience of continuous healing relationships*.

Relationships embrace and bridge the prevailing ethical theories. Therapeutic relationships are resources that help individuals create meaning for their situations and move them toward building trust for the future. They rely on methods of inquiry that include a consideration of the biological, emotional, behavioral, spiritual, social, cultural, and environmental layers of experience, which are interrelated. This is called a full relational context, and its elements provide continuous and reciprocal feedback to each other. Relational ethics assumes that individual action or behavior is shaped by a person's full relational context and cannot be understood outside it. This assumption would apply to the nurse, the patient, and the family.

Doherty (1991) has cogently described the core components of what might be described as the "ethical tradition" of mental health practice with which most nurses are familiar:

- Benevolence or caring, described as a disposition to enhance the welfare of the client and family as agents of their own lives.

- Justice, described as a disposition toward fair treatment of persons and groups, with special sensitivity to the vulnerable or disenfranchised.

- Courage, described as an ability to remain nonreactive in the face of tension, to face personal issues and to take risks for the welfare of the client and family.

- Truthfulness, described as the disposition toward honest expression of beliefs and a disinclination toward deception.

- Prudence, described as ability to balance competing needs and to act from reflection and consultation.

With its emphasis on trust building and on prevention, a relational ethic would add some components that are important elements of any relationship, but have special application to the asymmetrical relating that occurs in the health care system:

- Multidirected partiality, described as the simultaneous consideration of welfare of all the relating partners, especially those whose needs and interests might be in conflict.

- A periodic monitoring of the fairness in the relationship over time to identify patterns of unfairness (preventive interventions). Fairness here is defined as one person's responsible contribution to another.

- Deferring judgment or blame in the interests of trying to find common interests or a broader basis for action when the relationship gets stuck.

- Supporting moves toward an "I" position (asking or claiming one's own side; claiming a preference and clarifying expectations).

- Establishing an ongoing dialogue about consequences for relating partners.

- Acknowledging or crediting a relational partner's contributions to maintaining the balance of fairness in the relationship.

- Establishing forums in which ethical claims can be heard and worked out.

- Supporting and advocating for reasonable, reassuring, and caring leadership in environments that can sustain a relational ethic.

- Keeping destructive entitlement (invalid ethical claims for consideration) at the lowest possible levels by attending to justice issues.

- Creating opportunities for people to be contributors (building on assets).

- Teaching and implementing relational (many-sided) analysis of problems.

- Linking individual ethical action to common purpose (a team approach).

If openness to others and to their situation is the beginning of ethics, as is argued by philosophers whose work informs relational ethics, then we must address any and all barriers to that openness as it is lived (or not lived) within the immediacy and complexity of practice. If, as has been also argued, that disengagement and detachment are the source of malfeasance within health care systems, addressing such barriers is particularly urgent (Austin, 2011).

Because no one person can ever be the measure of the whole of any relational situation, the focus of relational ethics is not only the "autonomous" patients with rights, but anyone who might be affected by an action or event. Ethical conflicts are seen as opportunities for building trust. The methodology relies heavily on the professional's capacity for openness, directness, ethical sensitivity, and multidirected caring. The skills that are required are those of therapeutic resource and guide who seeks solutions in shared decision-making. This is in distinction to the expert who attempts to fix problems in isolation of context. Too often professionals, in evaluating the ethics of behavior and action, react to the signal and do not attend to the meaning of the signal within the larger context.

A relational conceptualization of the moral agent places increased emphasis on the asymmetries (inequities in strength, station, authority, power, resources, responsibility, status, and material, and physical or emotional contributions to the relationship) that naturally occur in therapeutic relationships. Reactivity, blame, and avoidance are viewed as signals of ethical distress in the relationship rather than as individual problems to be solved. Common ground is achieved through greater and greater explication of all sides in an ethical dilemma. Ethical sensitivity is acquired through mutually respectful engagement with those who might be affected by a decision or action. The consequences of action and behavior are shared among all relating partners. The requirements of relationship continue even when roles shift and functions change.

Fostering Mutually Respectful Relationships: Ethical Sensitivity and Mindfulness

Psychiatric-mental health nurses are indeed privileged to enter the world of other people's close relationships. They have learned about courage, risk taking, power, and control and that often people do harm to others not for any profound reasons, but just because they can. The families and communities they serve are living laboratories for understanding how relationships are maintained by compromises among expectations, aspirations, constraints, and obligations of its members. Their ethical sensitivities are built upon their experiences of relationship, and their practice informs them that ethical dilemmas arise in relationships and not solely within individuals.

The dialogues that psychiatric-mental health nurses have with each other are revealing of how their roots in relationship run deep. In a recent online discussion group among psychiatric nurses, a nursing student asked about the following situation that she encountered at her clinical site:

Case Study 13.2

I recently read about a patient's unfortunate experience in a hospital in which the patient over-heard some staff nurses making fun of the behavior of the psychiatric patients admitted into the unit. As I thought more about this issue, I realized that I had experienced this several times myself during my clinical rotations as a student nurse. I felt uncomfortable with this behavior, and I was wondering if there were any suggestions or resources available on how to address this issue as it happens? Also, what are some effective techniques that your facilities use to decrease the stigma of mental illness? (APNA all-purpose discussion forum, posted 9-01-2011)

The following are among a number of postings by nurses and nurse educators who were responding to the student's concern. They reveal how relationships shape a discussion of ethics without ever naming the discussion as being "about ethics."

> *One of the things that I believe we must take into consideration regarding how we discharge our emotions is that one in four persons are affected by mental illness—this means that one in four of our colleagues are personally affected as well. We all know better than to "vent" about issues related to race—at least we know better than doing so when persons of such race are in the nursing station with us. But mental illness cannot be seen the way race can, and we do not know who among us, of our colleagues—maybe even the ones we are "venting" to—may be personally affected by mental illness. When we do this, we not only perpetuate the stigma of those we treat, we add to the personal shame of those who work alongside us. Any one of us, or any one of our colleagues, or our family members or theirs, could very easily be the next person admitted to the unit where we work. Let's strive to be proud to serve them, should the need arise. (APNA all-purpose discussion forum, posted 9-04-2011)"*

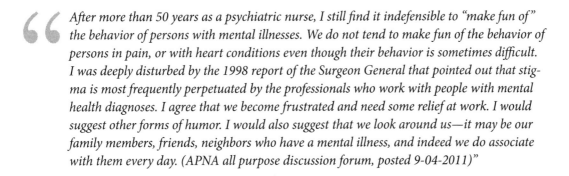

After more than 50 years as a psychiatric nurse, I still find it indefensible to "make fun of" the behavior of persons with mental illnesses. We do not tend to make fun of the behavior of persons in pain, or with heart conditions even though their behavior is sometimes difficult. I was deeply disturbed by the 1998 report of the Surgeon General that pointed out that stigma is most frequently perpetuated by the professionals who work with people with mental health diagnoses. I agree that we become frustrated and need some relief at work. I would suggest other forms of humor. I would also suggest that we look around us—it may be our family members, friends, neighbors who have a mental illness, and indeed we do associate with them every day. (APNA all purpose discussion forum, posted 9-04-2011)"

I want to be as respectful and provide the best care but, realistically, some of my patients use foul language directed at staff all day. Nurses are not saints, and sometimes you just have to go in the back room and vent. My first day in psych, I had a patient call me a name I can't even write here. Raised very strictly and not used to this language, I ran in the back room crying and thinking how could she call me that, what did I do wrong? A seasoned nurse told me swearing is common and to let it roll off of me like water and to not take it in and hurt me. (APNA all-purpose discussion forum, posted 9-02-2011)"

I spend a great deal of time working with my students on removing, deleting and avoiding stigma at all costs. I realize our staff members need to debrief and de-stress. Inpatient units can be amazingly stressful and challenging. And yet, I do not advocate the use of negative, caustic humor just so one individual can feel good about himself or herself. The point is: at what cost? For me, such an approach is never justifiable. The language we use and the way we decompress is a vital component of who we are as nurses, as individuals and as professionals. Is not our goal to promote recovery and hope of our patients? How can negative, demeaning humor be a part of that goal? (APNA all-purpose discussion forum, posted 9-06-2011)"

Listening to the voices of psychiatric-mental health nurses, we find it's clear that, whatever their practice domain, they live in a world of relationships, and these relationships give rise to conflicts. Many relational issues are embedded in the larger question of "stigma." They might include a stressful and challenging environment, few opportunities to debrief, lack of attention to preventive interventions, missed teaching and learning opportunities about respect and due consideration, personal characteristics of staff and patients, lack of support for learning and applying relational skills, lack of clarity about accountability, and stagnant leadership. These issues do not negate, but rather coexist with biopsychosocial treatment and interventions.

Apart from judging the ethical merit of any individual position on stigma considered in isolation, each of the nurses who posted comments, including the student, reflects a different vantage point. From the perspective of relational ethics, each vantage point merits consideration and each has to be addressed. The ethical task is to be open to hearing all of these vantage points, because they are embedded in multiple relationships that are connected to each other. Relational ethics would ask the "relational" questions as opposed to the "should and ought" questions.

PURPOSE EXERCISE: CONSIDER AND WRITE YOUR ANSWERS TO THE FOLLOWING QUESTIONS

1. What are the issues?

2. How are people positioned around the issues?

3. What are my responsibilities in this situation (my "I" position)?

4. What are the effects, and who will be affected by my actions?

5. What ethical standards and professional practices apply?

Psychiatric nurses practice in multiple settings that give rise to ethical conflicts that can be addressed through relationship. Again, the voices of psychiatric-mental health nurses are revealing:

Case Study 13.3

Therapists who may come into the home to do therapy may find themselves being drawn into a "friendship" type of relationship with their clients and families. They may feel the pressure of being asked personal questions about their own lives, given small gifts for holidays and special occasions, being offered the use of shore homes for vacations and weekends. This actually did happen to me with a client. A 57-year-old married woman who was estranged from her two daughters did not understand what she had done that "was so bad." She began to attempt to draw me into her family and asked personal questions about mine. She would attempt to give me small gifts and also offered me the use of her condo at the shore. At the same time, a nursing assistant who was helping her with personal care left, and the client started telling me about her private life. I used this opportunity to process why health care workers and therapists should not be sharing personal information with clients and how this impacted negatively on her own care. She had already been through quite a few nursing assistants before this. (J. Roman, personal communication, August 30, 2011)

In meeting the ethical challenge, the nurse might consider the following questions:

- How can all of the key relationships, including the relationship to the therapist, be best understood?

- From whose vantage point should ethical implications be considered?

- Who needs to be engaged in decision-making?

- Is there a forum for the nurse to exchange views on boundary issues with other colleagues?

Case Study 13.4

I received a call from a 60-year-old woman whose 38-year-old son was living with her and was a burden more than anything. He used drugs, had no job, and was verbally abusive toward her. He carried a diagnosis of bipolar disorder and saw a therapist and a psychiatrist, but would not adhere to a medication treatment regimen. She called me to talk about him and wanted me to come and see him for therapy. I told her that I could not see him unless he entered into a contract with me to be seen. She called me again and continued to talk about him on the phone. At one point, he got on the phone and I explained to him, as well as to her again, that I could only talk to him if he agreed to therapy. I finally was able to have her agree to be seen, so that I could help her deal with the situation. It was a continual challenge to have her talk about her own issues and not his. (J. Roman, personal communication, August 30, 2011)

In meeting the ethical challenge, the nurse might consider some guidelines from relational theory and therapy:

- Focus on facts *and* feelings.

- Focus on what is going on between people rather than inside them.

- Have some operating ethical principles to guide your thinking.

- Focus on process, not cause.

- Maintain flexibility.

- Try taking no position. Instead, consider both actions instead of one or the other.

Case Study 13.5

John, aged 16 years, lived with his mother and two siblings in a low income housing unit. He was truant from school and was being treated for substance abuse. He was constantly in difficulty with the police for theft and street fighting. John's mother had never married, and her children had different fathers. She was illiterate and in the course of her life had been exploited by males who later abandoned her. Neighbors also took advantage of her childlike need to please people in order to be cared about. Her behavior was characterized by helplessness, anger, depression, suspiciousness, and combativeness toward others. In the course of working with John and his family, it became clear that John responded to his mother's helplessness with aggressive, acting-out behavior toward others. As a family therapist, I understood that his behavior was his attempt to advocate for his mother in the only way he thought he could be effective. While his behavior expressed a lack of concern for himself or society, it also signaled his overriding concern to obtain justice for her."(Case files of Margaret Cotroneo)

Ignoring justice issues increases the entitlement of a relating partner and weakens the commitment to healing. Destructive entitlement is a claim for justice or fairness acted out in a substitute context, with little or no consideration of consequences for others. It produces disintegration of long-term relationships because the claims, though psychologically understood, are ethically invalid.

Ethical distress among nurses has been linked to concerns that arise not from within individuals, but from actions and considerations that occur between individuals: appropriateness of treatment choices, patient autonomy, interpersonal relationships among professionals and with the family (being caught in the middle), patient suffering, colliding expectations of health care professionals, institutional obstacles, and poor communication (Pavlish, Brown-Saltzman, Hersh, Shirk, & Nudelman, 2011). These elements of distress are the fruits of complex and dynamic relational systems in action. Multiple boundary issues can be added to the list. In other words, the very nature of the nurse-patient-family relationship with all of its asymmetries gives rise to ethical conflicts.

These asymmetries are in the nature of a "therapeutic relationship" and are well described in the clinical literature across disciplines. Asymmetries often present as colliding expectations, and they are a frequent source of frustration and confusion for psychiatric-mental health nurses. Ethics in a transforming practice environment requires ethical sensitivity, mindfulness, and a heavy dose of moral courage. This poses a creative challenge to nursing leadership to create environments that incorporate the development of ethical sensitivity and mindfulness into clinical practice across settings.

Conclusion

We have moved into another of those rather confusing periods of our global history in which some are afflicted by "choice and change fatigue," while others must live in the narrow space to which they are confined by few choices and changes that are too slow to prevent death and disability. The ethical challenge for psychiatric-mental health nurses is to widen the circle of "quality of life" for those we serve, so that precious human resources can be sustained while we participate in transforming our health care system. The ethics of choice will drive health policy and practice well into the future. In this milieu, the "autonomous person" in isolation of a relevant context will no longer exist as an ethical norm (IOM, 2011, pp. 576-577). Rather, the ethical norm will be the sustained relationships built on reciprocity, trust, and social justice. Therapeutic relationship has deep roots in psychiatric-mental health nursing, whose practitioners are generally educated to counsel and communicate with patients and families more frequently and to work across disciplinary boundaries to better care for them. The relational core of psychiatric-mental health nursing practice provides a solid foundation for meeting the needs for prevention; care coordination; patient, family, and community-centered care; and collaborative care that are driving a transforming health care system.

Talk About It!

- With the development of new evidence-based practices and emerging technologies such as telemedicine, what kind of support and guidance do you need to sustain the commitment to a therapeutic relationship?

- Do you have an ethical framework that prepares you to think preventatively about ethical dilemmas?

- When you are pressed for time and must deal with complicated clinical dilemmas, do you have strategies that help you to be aware and alert to the consequences of your interventions for all those who might be affected?

- Think about your personal values that shape your ethical responses in therapeutic relationships. What guides you when the client's or their family's values and ethics are in conflict with your own?

References

American Psychiatric Nurses Association and the International Society of Psychiatric-Mental Health Nurses. (2007). *Psychiatric–Mental health nursing scope and standards of practice.* Silver Spring, MD: American Nurses Publishing.

Austin, W. (2011). *Engagement in contemporary practice: A relational ethics perspective.* Retrieved from http://www.scielo.br/scielo.php?script=sci_arttext&pid=S0104-07072006000500015&lng=en&nrm=iso or http://dx.doi.org/10.1590/S0104-07072006000500015

Cotroneo, M., Kurlowicz, L. H., Outlaw, F. H., Burgess, A. W., & Evans, L. K. (2001). Psychiatric-mental health nursing at the interface: Revisioning education for the specialty. *Issues in Mental Health Nursing, 22*(5), 549-69.

Diez Rouz, A. V. (2011, July 21). Complex systems thinking may help us transcend current impasses in health disparities research. *American Journal of Public Health.* [Published online ahead of print]. doi: 10.2105/AJPH.2011.300149

Doherty, W. J. (1991). Virtue ethics: The person of the therapist. Ethics. Not just black and white. *Newsletter of the American Family Therapy Academy, 46,* 19-21.

Epstein, R., & Street, R. (2011). Shared mind: Communication, decision-making and autonomy in serious illness. *Annals of Family Medicine, 9*(5), 454-461.

Harrowing, J. N., Mill, J., Spiers, J., Kulig, J., & Kipp, W. (2010). Culture, context and community: Ethical considerations for global nursing research. *International Nursing Review, 57*(1), 70-77.

Institute of Medicine (IOM). (1988). *The future of public health.* Washington, DC: National Academies Press.

Institute of Medicine (IOM). (1996). *Primary care: America's health in a new era.* Washington, DC: The National Academies Press.

Institute of Medicine (IOM). (2001). *Crossing the quality chasm: A new health system for the 21ˢᵗ century.* Washington, DC: The National Academies Press.

Institute of Medicine (IOM). (2003). *Unequal treatment: Confronting racial and ethnic disparities in health care.* Washington, DC: The National Academies Press.

Institute of Medicine (IOM). (2011). *The future of nursing: Leading change, advancing health.* Washington, DC: The National Academies Press

International Council of Nurses (ICN). (2006). *Code of ethics for nurses.* Geneva, Switzerland: Author.

Kessler, R. C., Chiu, W. T., Demler, O., Merikangas, K. R., & Walters, E. E. (2005). Prevalence, severity, and comorbidity of 12-month DSM-IV disorders in the National Comorbidity Survey Replication. *Archives General Psychiatry, 62*(6), 617–27.

Kiecolt-Glaser, J. K., & Glaser, R. (1986). Psychological influences on immunity. *Psychosomatics, 27*(9), 621-624.

Lambert, T. W., Soskolne, C. L., Bergum, V., Howell, J., Dossetor, J. B. (2003). Ethical perspectives for public and environmental health: Fostering autonomy and the right to know. *Environmental Health Perspectives, 111*(2), 133-137.

McDaniel, S. H., Campbell, T. L., Hepworth, J., & Lorenz, A. (2005). *Family-oriented primary care* (2nd ed.). New York: Springer.

National Institute of Mental Health (NIMH). (2011, Sept. 6). No health without mental health. *Director's blog.* Retrieved from http://www.nimh.nih.gov/about/director/2011/no-health-without-mental-health.shtml

National Prevention Council. (2011). National prevention strategy. U.S. Department of Health and Human Services, Office of the Surgeon General. Retrieved from http://www. healthcare.gov/prevention/nphpphc/strategy/report

The Patient Protection and Affordable Care Act, P.L. 111-148. (2010, March 23). *HealthCare.gov.* Retrieved from www.healthcare.gov/law/full/

Pavlish, C., Brown-Saltzman, K., Hersh, M., Shirk, M., & Nudelman, O. (2011). Early indicators and risk for ethical issues in clinical practice. *Journal of Nursing Scholarship, 43*(1), 13-21.

Peplau, H. E. (1952). Interpersonal Relations in Nursing. New York: G. P. Putnam & Sons.

Pettersen, T. (2011). The ethics of care: Normative structures and empirical implications. *Health Care Analysis, 19*(1), 51-64.

Registered Psychiatric Nurses of Canada. (2010). *Code of ethics & standards of psychiatric nursing practice.* Edmonton, Alberta: Author.

Reich, R. B. (2009). *Relational capital.* Washington Speakers Bureau, Alexandria, Virginia. Retrieved from www.WashingtonSpeakers.com

Seaburn, D. B, McDaniel, S. H., Kim, S. & Bassen, D. (2005). The role of the family in resolving bioethical dilemmas: Clinical insights from a family systems perspective. *Journal of Clinical Ethics, 15*(2), 123-134.

Thomas, J. C., & Young, S. (2011, Sept. 22). Wake me up when there's a crisis: Progress on state pandemic influenza ethics preparedness. *American Journal of Public Health.* [Published ahead of print]. Retrieved from http://ajph.aphapublications.org/cgi/content/abstract/AJPH.2011.300293v1

Ulrich, C. M., Hamric, A. B., & Grady, C. (2010). Moral distress: A growing problem in the health professions? *Hastings Center Report, 40*(1), 20-22.

INDEX

N

O–P

T

teamwork, colleagues, 40

technology

advanced illness care and, 8–9

EHRs (electronic health records), 10–11

preventive measures, 11–12

end-of-life and, 8–9

future of nursing care and, 7–8

relationship changes, 206–207

technological imperative, 169–170

Texas abuse of power, nurses and, 46–47

Thalidomide, 106

The Silent Treatment, 41

TJC (The Joint Commission), behaviors undermining patient safety, 41

To Err Is Human, 40

trust

in nurses, 38

relationships and, 203

truth-telling, errors and, 176–177

Tuskegee Study of Untreated Syphilis in Black Men, 105

U

undiscussable situations, 46

unintentional injury to children, 186

V

virtues in long-term care, 139

virtues-based model of decision-making, 27–28

vulnerable populations, genetic testing, 88–89

W–X–Y–Z

Walker, Margaret Urban, ethics of responsibility, 134

WHO (World Health Organization), core competencies, 12

withdrawal *versus* withholding, 171–172

workforce, health care, aging issues, 5–7